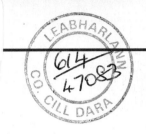
100 Questions & Answers About Childhood Immunizations

Thomas H. Belhorn, MD, PhD

University of North Carolina
North Carolina Children's Hospital
Pediatrics–Infectious Diseases
Chapel Hill, North Carolina

JONES AND BARTLETT PUBLISHERS
Sudbury, Massachusetts
BOSTON   TORONTO   LONDON   SINGAPORE

World Headquarters

Jones and Bartlett Publishers
40 Tall Pine Drive
Sudbury, MA 01776
978-443-5000
info@jbpub.com
www.jbpub.com

Jones and Bartlett Publishers
Canada
6339 Ormindale Way
Mississauga, Ontario L5V 1J2
Canada

Jones and Bartlett Publishers
International
Barb House, Barb Mews
London W6 7PA
United Kingdom

Jones and Bartlett's books and products are available through most bookstores and online booksellers. To contact Jones and Bartlett Publishers directly, call 800-832-0034, fax 978-443-8000, or visit our website, www.jbpub.com.

Substantial discounts on bulk quantities of Jones and Bartlett's publications are available to corporations, professional associations, and other qualified organizations. For details and specific discount information, contact the special sales department at Jones and Bartlett via the above contact information or send an email to specialsales@jbpub.com.

The authors, editor, and publisher have made every effort to provide accurate information. However, they are not responsible for errors, omissions, or for any outcomes related to the use of the contents of this book and take no responsibility for the use of the products and procedures described. Treatments and side effects described in this book may not be applicable to all people; likewise, some people may require a dose or experience a side effect that is not described herein. Drugs and medical devices are discussed that may have limited availability controlled by the Food and Drug Administration (FDA) for use only in a research study or clinical trial. Research, clinical practice, and government regulations often change the accepted standard in this field. When consideration is being given to use of any drug in the clinical setting, the healthcare provider or reader is responsible for determining FDA status of the drug, reading the package insert, and reviewing prescribing information for the most up-to-date recommendations on dose, precautions, and contraindications, and determining the appropriate usage for the product. This is especially important in the case of drugs that are new or seldom used.

Production Credits

Executive Publisher: Christopher Davis
Associate Editor: Kathy Richardson
Sr. Editorial Assistant: Jessica Acox
Production Director: Amy Rose
Production Editor: Daniel Stone
Associate Marketing Manager: Ilana Goddess

V.P., Manufacturing and Inventory Control:
   Therese Connell
Cover Design: Kristin E. Ohlin
Composition: Spoke & Wheel/Jason Miranda
Printing and Binding: Malloy, Inc.
Cover Printing: Malloy, Inc.

Cover Credits
Cover Image: Top Left: © Dana Bartekoske/ShutterStock, Inc.; Top Right: © iofoto/ShutterStock, Inc.;
   Bottom: © Sonya Etchison/ShutterStock, Inc.

Library of Congress Cataloging-in-Publication Data
Belhorn, Thomas H.
   100 questions & answers about childhood immunizations / Thomas H. Belhorn
      p. cm.
   Includes bibliographical references and index.
   ISBN-13: 978-0-7637-5497-6
   ISBN-10: 0-7637-5497-8
   1. Immunization of children—Miscellanea. 2. Vaccination of children—Miscellanea. I. Title. II. Title: One
   hundred questions and answers about childhood immunizations. III. Title: 100 questions and answers about
   childhood immunizations.
   RJ240.B45 2009
   614.4'7083—dc22
                          2008029364

6048

Printed in the United States of America
12 11 10 09 08   10 9 8 7 6 5 4 3 2 1

I wish to give special thanks to my family, especially Linda, Chris, and Stephanie, for their continued love and support.

I dedicate this book to all the teachers in my family who inspired me with their dedication and passion as educators of school children. For Aunt Kay and Uncle Jack, Aunt Jean, and especially my mother, Anne Belhorn—may your footsteps continue to be my guide.

CONTENTS

Do I believe in vaccines?

I will be the first to admit that I am biased due to my profession as a pediatric infectious disease specialist. It is my job to help with the diagnosis and management of children with a spectrum of challenging, unusual, or severe infections. As many vaccine preventable diseases are now rare, I am often the doctor seeing children who may or do have a vaccine-preventable disease.

Personal experiences help solidify belief. My first encounter as a physician with a new vaccine was with a conjugate vaccine for *Haemophilus influenzae*. I was a resident in pediatrics from 1987 to 1990. During my first year in residency I helped provide care to many children, most of them infants and very young children, with severe infections (including meningitis, epiglottitis, periorbital cellulitis, and others) due to the bacterium *Haemophilus influenzae*. Although many children recovered, some did not. The new conjugate vaccine for this bacterium then became part of the recommended immunization schedule for infants. By the end of my residency, I had witnessed an amazing change— the disappearance of severe infections caused by this bacterium. There were no more admissions of children with epiglottitis, and I no longer saw children with this type of meningitis—infections due to this type of bacteria practically vanished. I was an eyewitness to the power of this vaccine, and I became a believer. For other vaccine-preventable infections the decreased frequency of disease has been due not only to vaccines but also to improvements in sanitation, hygiene, and other advances in public health—but in my opinion, vaccines have been the major factor.

Do vaccines always work? I wish I could say vaccines always work. I have had the dubious honor of being an infectious disease doctor who had influenza one year despite having had my annual vaccine earlier in the influenza season. I tried to convince myself that my illness was less severe since I received the vaccine, but of course that would be hard to prove. I will rejoice when one of my virology colleagues discovers an influenza vaccine effective against all strains of this virus. The varicella vaccine, likewise, does not always prevent chickenpox, and recent mumps outbreaks in individuals previously immunized with this vaccine have caused some concern.

Yet the efficacy of many vaccines is clearly excellent. It is easy to forget about some diseases when we no longer hear about them. Smallpox has been eradicated. Polio may soon be eradicated. I have cared for very few children with tetanus and measles in the United States, and all have been infants too young to be immunized or children who never received the vaccine. I have only experienced infections such as diphtheria as a medical missionary in an area of the world where vaccines are not well utilized. It is clear to me that vaccines have made a tremendous positive impact in decreasing childhood diseases.

Are vaccines safe? No medicine, or vaccine, is totally without risk. Even medicines such as aspirin, acetaminophen (Tylenol), and common over-the-counter medicines have side effects which can be serious in a small number of children. Vaccines are no different, but in my opinion the benefits for most vaccines far outweigh the risks. Many issues regarding vaccine safety are discussed in this book.

A mother once told me that a great question to ask your child's pediatrician was whether or not they give all the recommended vaccines to their own children. I think that is an excellent question. I am a father. I try to weigh the risks and benefits of everything given to my own children, and the decision is not automatic. If I have concerns of safety, they do not receive that medication. But over the years I have decided, after careful consideration, to fully immunize my own children as recommended by the current immunization schedule. I have had the luxury of being able to follow vaccine development and clinical trials long before a vaccine is approved for use in children, allowing me to judge for myself whether it is safe and effective. I can not guarantee I will always be able to say this, but I do recommend and use the currently-recommended vaccines for my own children and my own patients.

My goal in writing this book is not to convince the reader that any specific viewpoint is right or that they should or should not give vaccines to their children. Instead, I hope I have chosen questions and provided answers to help explain the basic information needed to understand some of the issues involved with this decision. Further information can be obtained from your child's health care provider and other resources as needed to help with these decisions.

I am eternally grateful to the many children, families, and fellow healthcare providers who have impacted so many areas of my life during my professional career. I am especially privileged to work with so many individuals at North Carolina Children's Hospital and The University of North Carolina in Chapel Hill who continually exemplify the greatest level of expertise and compassion in the care they provide for children. Lastly I am grateful to Jones and Bartlett Publishers for asking me to write this book; it has been a pleasure to write and I hope it will bring enjoyment and further knowledge to the reader.

Thomas H. Belhorn, MD, PhD

Patient Biographies

Mary Ellen is a 40-year veteran of the clinical microbiology laboratory at UNC Health Care who has volunteered as a laboratory assistant for the medical technology program at UNC. She loves to teach, and she loves bacteria.

Amy Lynn Kelley is the mother of five children (ages 2 years–10 years) and is the Children's Pastor at Newhope Church in Durham, NC. She hopes this book will be helpful to parents and is thankful for the medical community for all they do for kids today!

Abby is a high school senior who will be attending UNC–Chapel Hill in the fall. She plans on majoring in chemistry and having a future career in medicine. She enjoys playing the flute and listening to music in her free time.

PART ONE

The Basics

What is a vaccine?

What do "immunity" and "immunization" mean?

How do vaccines work?

More . . .

1. What is a vaccine?

A **vaccine** is a substance that teaches the body to recognize and defend itself against a disease-causing germ. Good nutrition, sleep, good hygiene, and many other things are so important for your child's health, but a vaccine is unique—it is given to prepare your child's body to fight off a specific germ or disease. Although vaccines provide many benefits, which will be discussed in other sections of this book, the main purpose of giving a vaccine to your child is to help keep your child healthy.

Childhood infections are caused by a large number of germs, or **microorganisms**—things too small to be seen by the naked eye which may cause infections. Many common childhood infections are caused by one of two types of germs, bacteria or viruses. These microorganisms are widespread in the environment as well as throughout your child's body. **Bacteria** are single-cell organisms that get nourishment from the environment. Normally, large numbers of bacteria live in and on your body, often performing useful and necessary functions; but certain types of bacteria can cause disease. **Viruses** differ from bacteria in that they are usually considered "non-living." Viruses need to live in other cells to survive. Because of this difference, most bacteria can be killed by medicines called antibiotics, but these drugs have no effect on viruses.

A vaccine has to be introduced into the body, usually by a shot, to start the process which builds up protection against the germ. Because a vaccine is designed to protect from disease without causing the disease, the normal live bacterium or wild type virus is not what is used in a vaccine. Instead, each vaccine contains a different form of the microorganism which is chosen specifically for its ability to stimulate the body to build up protection

without actually giving the disease. There are four tra-
ditional forms, or types of vaccines, as listed below:

- Killed microorganisms
- Live, attenuated (weakened) microorganisms
- **Toxoids** (inactive toxic compounds)
- **Subunit vaccine** (has only a part of the
  microorganism)

The active part of the vaccine can be combined with
other substances to make it more effective in creating
a protective response in your child. Further details on
types of vaccines and additives to vaccines are provided
in other sections of this book.

2. What do "immunity" and "immunization" mean?

A short definition of **immunity** is protection from disease. If you are protected from a disease and are no longer
susceptible to its effects, you are immune, or have immunity against that specific illness. The process of giving a
vaccine to someone in order to bring about immunity is
called **immunization**, or **vaccination**.

Children have several types of immunity. All children are
born with **natural (or innate) immunity**, which provides
general protection against certain germs. This protection
is non-specific and is part of the general response your
child's body has to the presence of an invading germ.
Your child's skin, stomach lining, nose, sinuses, and
other body surfaces all help provide this natural immunity by creating a barrier against many germs. Certain
body fluids or secretions, and other parts of the immune
system also provide a non-specific response to protect

Toxoids

Types of vaccines
which are made
from inactive toxic
compounds.

Subunit vaccine

One of the four
basic types of vac-
cines. It is named
"subunit" because
only part of the
microorganism
is present in the
vaccine.

Immunity

Protection of the
body from either
a disease or from
infection by a
microorganism.

**Immunization/
Vaccination**

The process of giving
a vaccine to some-
one in order to bring
about immunity.

**Natural immunity/
Innate immunity**

Part of the general
response of the body
to the presence of an
invading germ which
provides non-specific
protection.

Active (Adaptive) immunity

Protection of the body against disease or infection due to specific microorganisms.

A short definition of immunity is protection from disease.

Passive immunity

Protection of the body from disease or infection which develops when a person is given antibodies.

Antibodies

Proteins made by immune cells in the body which help the body recognize microorganisms and fight off infection.

Immune system

The cells, glands, and fluids throughout the body which work together to fight microorganisms.

against germs. **Active**, or **adaptive**, **immunity** occurs throughout your life, after either natural infections or immunization with vaccines. After infection or immunization, the body learns to recognize a specific microorganism and creates memory cells to help protect the body against future infections with the same or similar germs. It is true that natural infection often creates longer lasting immunity than vaccines. However, with natural infection you risk having a significant illness or disease, which for some infections can cause severe complications or death. Lastly, there is **passive immunity**, which develops when a person is given **antibodies** to help fight off infections. Passive immunity is important in infants. Antibodies are passed across the placenta to the baby, especially in the third trimester of pregnancy, and babies who are breast fed get additional protection from the mother's breast milk to help fight infections. Unfortunately, passive immunity does not last long; whereas, active immunity can be lifelong. All of these forms of immunity combine to help protect your child from infections.

Your child has a unique **immune system** which is very different from everyone else's immune system. In addition, the degree of immunity or protection your child has against specific diseases will be different from your own immunity and from that possessed by other children. It is often difficult to understand why some children seem to be very healthy and rarely suffer from infectious diseases, while others seem to be sick frequently and to have more severe or longer duration of symptoms with the same infection. How well your child's immune system functions depends on genetics (factors inherited from parents), general health and nutrition, degree and extent of exposure to microorganisms, prior infections, vaccine history, and many other factors. Luckily, as children age, they do develop immunity to more germs and usually have less frequent infections.

3. How do vaccines work?

When your child is infected by a germ to which he is susceptible, the germs start to multiply, or reproduce, in the body. Healthy children have a complete immune system composed of cells, glands, and fluids throughout their bodies which work together to fight germs. The job of the immune system is to react to the germs to help fight the infection. The process is quite complex, but involves recognizing the germ as foreign and producing compounds called antibodies, which are germ-specific and help fight the infection. As part of this process, your child's immune system develops memory cells for that germ. The next time your child encounters the same virus or bacterium, these memory cells are activated and attack the germ quickly, usually preventing your child from becoming ill from the infection. This entire process is called the development of immunity.

Vaccines are designed to do the same thing by mimicking the natural infection without the risk of having the disease or illness. Since vaccines are made from the same weakened germs, or parts or products from the germ, the immune system "practices" fighting the disease by making antibodies that recognize specific parts of the germ, just as they do in the natural infection. The same memory cells are made, and when your child is exposed to the wild type virus or bacterium later, the memory cells are activated and work to prevent your child from getting sick from the infection. Therefore, your child gets the immunity, or protection, from the disease without having the risk of the signs and symptoms of the actual disease.

4. How are vaccines made?

Before a vaccine can be developed, scientists must have a good understanding of the virus or bacterium, especially how it causes disease. Only then can an intelligent decision be made how to prevent infection or prevent the disease caused by the organism and how to best create a vaccine which will be safe and effective.

Vaccines can be made in several different ways. There have traditionally been four types of vaccines used in children. **Killed vaccines** contain microorganisms that have been killed, or inactivated, usually by heat or chemicals. These vaccines cannot cause disease in the recipient; but, since they are not living, several doses of vaccine are often required to produce a good immune response. Live **attenuated**, or weakened, **vaccines** are made by changing some component of the germ, usually in the process of growing the microorganism, so that it loses the properties that made it virulent, or capable of causing disease. Sometimes a related microorganism which gives the same immunity but cannot cause the same disease can be used in the vaccine. Live vaccines often give an immune response of longer duration than killed vaccines, but they may carry a risk of causing a mild form of the disease. In a healthy child, this illness is much less severe compared with illness associated with the usual infection; however, a child who has a weak immune system can still experience a serious illness. Therefore, live attenuated vaccines are sometimes contraindicated in people with certain diseases of the immune system or those taking medications which weaken the immune system.

A third type of vaccine is one consisting of a toxoid, which is an inactivated toxin/toxic substance produced by the organism. Some microorganisms cause diseases

Killed vaccines

Vaccines which contain only killed or inactivated microorganisms.

Attenuated vaccines

Vaccines which contain live but weakened microorganisms.

by producing a toxin, and the best protection from disease is helping the body to become immune to the toxin. A fourth vaccine type is a subunit vaccine. In this type of vaccine, only a part of the microorganism is used to make the vaccine, rather than the whole organism. Neither toxoid vaccines nor subunit vaccines can give the vaccine recipient disease.

Some vaccines have another compound attached to the microorganism, or its part, to create a better immune response. This is called a **conjugate vaccine**.

After a candidate vaccine is produced, it must go through extensive testing to prove it is safe as well as effective in the population in which it is going to be used.

5. How effective are vaccines in preventing diseases?

Vaccines vary in effectiveness at preventing diseases. Most vaccines are very effective, but some vaccines do not work all the time. **Smallpox** is the best example of an effective vaccine. Smallpox was a disease that killed millions of people every year, but the worldwide vaccination program using this vaccine wiped out smallpox. It was the first disease, and so far the only one, to be completely eradicated by the use of a vaccine. There have been many other tremendous successes in vaccines. **Polio** has been eradicated from the western hemisphere and efforts continue to completely eradicate it from the world. Diseases such as **diphtheria** and **measles** have been brought to very low levels in the United States. Table I shows some of the successes in fighting infectious diseases in the United States in the vaccine era.

Conjugate vaccine

A vaccine which has the microorganism (or part of the microorganism) attached to another compound which creates a better immune response.

Smallpox

A disease characterized by high fever, spots in the mouth, and a rash with classic "pox" lesions.

Polio

The disease caused by the virus of the same name.

Diphtheria

The disease caused by the bacterium *Corynebacterium diphtheriae*.

Measles

The disease caused by the virus of the same name.

Table 1 Impact of Vaccines on Ten Infectious Diseases in the United States

Year Vaccine Developed and/or Licensed	Disease/Vaccine	Disease Impact Before Introduction of Vaccine (United States)	Disease Impact After Introduction of Vaccine— 2006 Data (United States)
1797 (not widely used before 1900)	Smallpox	In 1900, 21,064 reported cases, 894 deaths	Disease eradicated in 1977
1923	Diphtheria	In 1920, 147,991 reported cases, 13,170 deaths	0
1926	Pertussis	In 1922, 107,474 reported cases, 5099 deaths	15,632 cases
1927	Tetanus	In early-mid 1920s, 1300 cases per year	41 cases
1955	Polio	Between 1951–1954, an average of 16,316 cases reported, 1879 deaths	Wild-type polio eradicated in Western Hemisphere in 1991
1963	Measles	Between 1958–1962, an average of 503,282 cases reported, 432 deaths	55 cases
1967	Mumps	In 1964, 212,000 cases	6584 cases
1969	Rubella	In 1964–1965, epidemic with average 20,000 infants born with congenital rubella syndrome, 2100 neonatal deaths, 11,250 miscarriages	11 cases of rubella, only one case of congenital rubella
1982	Hepatitis B	In 1982, 22,177 cases reported	4713 cases
1985	Haemophilus influenzae type b	Estimated 20,000 cases per year prior to vaccine	29 cases

Table modified from AAP Childhood Immunization Support Program; source of data used in modification from Centers for Disease Control and Prevention, Morbidity and Mortality Reports

Although most vaccines work about 90–100% of the time (some may be less effective), sometimes a specific vaccine will not work. The reasons for this are variable and depend on the vaccine as well as your child's immune system. Immunizing everyone in the family and in the community is important because it helps to decrease the risk that your child will get the illness from someone else. This is known as **herd immunity**. People who have been immunized are much less likely to spread infection to others, and therefore they help protect others from the spread of disease. Even people who have not received a vaccine can be protected by herd immunity, because they are less likely to be exposed to someone with a vaccine-preventable disease if enough people in the community have been immunized. Research has shown that, for some infections, about 95% of people in the community must be protected by the vaccine to achieve herd immunity.

Herd immunity

Protection of unimmunized people from a specific infection or disease which is obtained by immunizing a large percentage of people.

Today, many cases of rare diseases occur in the United States when non-immunized people get the disease after travel or contact with someone who has traveled to a country where the disease is still common. Unfortunately, that person can subsequently pass the disease on to other unimmunized people, to those too young to get vaccines, or to those for whom vaccines are contraindicated. With high immunization rates, herd immunity will enable even vaccines which are not 100% effective to slow the spread of infections and prevent large outbreaks of the disease.

Immunizing everyone in the family and in the community is important because it helps to decrease the risk that your child will get the illness from someone else.

Pertussis

The disease caused by infection with the bacterium *Bordetella pertussis*.

Chickenpox

An illness with fever and a characteristic rash.

Pneumococcus

Another name for the bacterium *Streptococcus pneumoniae*, a bacterium associated with many types of infections in children.

Tetanus

A disease which affects the nervous system and is caused by the bacterium *Clostridium tetani*. Also called "lockjaw."

Mumps

A disease caused by the mumps virus.

Tetanus is an example of a disease which we will always be at risk of acquiring because the bacterium lives in dirt and is not transmitted from person to person.

6. *Are vaccines still necessary since many diseases are now rare?*

The frequency of vaccine-preventable diseases still seen in the United States varies significantly with each disease/organism. Some diseases are still encountered frequently and not receiving a vaccine against them results in a significant risk of having an infection with that organism. Such diseases include **pertussis** (whooping cough), **chickenpox**, bacterial infections due to **pneumococcus**, and others. **Tetanus** is an example of a disease which we will always be at risk of acquiring because the bacterium lives in dirt and is not transmitted from person to person. Since we cannot get rid of this bacterium, there will always be a risk of getting the disease. Some diseases are still encountered in occasional outbreaks and individual cases. These include diseases like measles and **mumps**. Some diseases, such as polio and diphtheria, have been virtually eliminated in the United States but are still present in other nations. If an unimmunized person travels to these areas or is exposed to infected individuals from these areas, they are at risk of getting the infection and spreading the disease to other people. Many of our recent outbreaks of diseases, like measles, are associated with such exposures. Some of these diseases are rare in the United States only because we are immunizing our children against them.

History has already shown us what happens when immunization rates drop. In the 1970s, many people in Japan stopped immunizing their children against pertussis. In the five-year period when immunization rates dropped to only 10% of children receiving the vaccine, the rate of infections rose by more than 30-fold and deaths due to pertussis went from zero to 41 per year at the end of the five years. Reinstitution of the vaccine caused a reversal of the trend. Similar occurrences have happened in Great Britain with other vaccine-preventable diseases. Public health experts know that some diseases may never be eliminated, but there is hope of elimination for some vaccine-preventable diseases. It is important to keep immunizing our children for their improved health and the improved health of their children.

7. Can a vaccine give you the disease it is supposed to prevent?

Most childhood vaccines are either killed vaccines, subunit vaccines (containing only a part of the pathogen), or a toxoid (inactive toxin produced by the pathogen). The whole germ is not part of these vaccines, and there is nothing in the vaccines capable of making the germ or causing that disease. A few childhood vaccines are live, attenuated (weakened) virus vaccines. These vaccines are designed to reproduce in the body in a limited amount. The virus made in the body is of a type which has been changed to a weaker form which is unable to cause the original disease. Examples of the live vaccines include the current vaccines for measles, mumps, and rubella (in the **MMR vaccine**), the **varicella** (chickenpox) vaccine, and the rotavirus vaccine. Usually these vaccines do not make your child ill, but healthy children run a small risk of getting very mild symptoms similar to the original illness (e.g., mild diarrhea for **rotavirus**, mild rash for chickenpox or measles). Children with weakened immune systems also usually do well with these vaccines, but in theory could develop a worse disease with a live vaccine. Therefore, these vaccines are not to be given to children with certain types of immune deficiency or weakened immune systems.

MMR vaccine

The live virus vaccine given to prevent measles, mumps, and rubella.

Varicella

An illness with fever and a characteristic rash of pox on the skin.

Rotavirus

A common, highly contagious virus that is an important cause of severe diarrhea in children.

THE BASICS

8. How long will a vaccine protect my child from disease?

To some extent, the length of time your child is protected after an immunization can be predicted for a specific vaccine, but it is variable. The duration of immunity depends on the type of vaccine used, your child's immune system and immune response to the vaccine, the microorganism causing the infection, and even how frequently your child is exposed to the natural disease in the community. Some vaccines, for example the measles vaccine and hepatitis B vaccine, are known to create lifelong immunity in many people. Other vaccines, such as the vaccine for tetanus, produce immunity which decreases at a fairly predictable rate, and **booster doses** of vaccines are scheduled to make sure that adequate protection continues. The pertussis vaccine is another vaccine which does not produce lifelong immunity, and a booster dose is recommended during adolescence.

The vaccines against the **influenza** virus ("flu" virus) have always been a challenge to produce. As will be discussed in a later question, the immunity is fairly short-lived, plus the virus itself can change from year to year. Therefore, the current vaccine strategy for influenza is for scientists to make an educated guess about which strains of flu virus will cause infections the next year, create a vaccine against those strains of flu, and give this vaccine to people every fall to help prevent influenza infection.

If your child already has immunity against a specific infection, and he comes in contact with someone who has that infection, that exposure may actually boost his own immunity. Chickenpox is an example of a disease in which repeated exposures may help boost the immune system. The varicella vaccine (chickenpox vaccine) is

Booster doses

Additional doses of a vaccine given to increase the immunity provided by that vaccine.

Influenza

Often called "the flu," this is the disease caused by one of the influenza viruses.

The vaccines against the influenza virus ("flu" virus) have always been a challenge to produce.

routinely given to young children. Therefore, most children develop immunity against this virus either from the vaccine or from natural infection early in life. If your child is exposed to someone with chickenpox in later childhood, the virus exposure is less likely to cause disease but it may provide a boost to the immune system. This may also happen with other germs such as pertussis and other common childhood infections, and create situations where the duration of protection from vaccines is lengthened by exposures to others with that infectious disease.

Scientists often have difficulty predicting how long a specific vaccine will provide protection. Measuring how much antibody against the bacterium or virus is produced in the bloodstream after someone gets a vaccine is thought to be one measure of protection from disease. Therefore, clinical studies are often designed in which a group of people receives the vaccine, samples of blood are checked to measure the amount of specific antibody produced soon after immunization, and repeat blood samples are checked for antibody multiple times over several years. If the level of antibodies remains high for many years, the vaccine is thought to create long-term immunity. One problem, though, is that vaccines can produce different types of immunity, including memory cells, which are often harder to measure. For some infections, the amount of antibody in the blood is a good predictor of the amount of protection the person has against infection. But for other diseases, the antibody levels decrease, but the person is still protected. Therefore, long term monitoring of people who received the vaccine for evidence of infection or disease later in life is helpful in determining the duration of protection produced by a specific vaccine. Further information about how well vaccines work will be given in the sections on specific vaccines.

9. What else can I do to prevent infections and illnesses besides giving my children vaccines?

Good nutrition and a healthy lifestyle are crucial to keep your immune system healthy. Many minerals, vitamins, and other nutrients are needed by the cells, enzymes, and other parts of our immune system in order for it to work to fight off infections. Your children get these vital nutrients from the foods they eat. If your children eat a well-balanced diet with fresh fruits and vegetables, whole grains, and other nutritious foods, they will usually have an adequate supply of these vital nutrients. Unfortunately, the diets of many children in the United States consist of too many processed or "fast foods" which have less nutritional value. Obesity is currently a significant problem for many children in the United States. Surprisingly, these children are often malnourished because much of their diet consists of foods with poor nutritional value. If you are concerned about your child's diet and nutritional intake, you may wish to discuss with your child's doctor whether a multivitamin/mineral supplement would be of value for your child.

In addition to good nutrition, maintaining a healthy lifestyle is very important to your child's immune system.

In addition to good nutrition, maintaining a healthy lifestyle is very important to your child's immune system. Think about whether your children get enough rest and sleep. Are they staying fit and getting enough exercise? Do they have a lot of stress in their lives, and have you taught them how to reduce stress? All of these factors have been linked to the health of the immune system. Tobacco and drug use have adverse effects on immunity. Even secondhand smoke (exposure to tobacco smoke) has been shown to increase children's risk of respiratory infections. Good attention to your child's oral health, making sure they brush their teeth and see a dentist regularly, is beneficial for overall good health. All of these healthy lifestyle choices should be taught to your children and are, of course, best learned if the parent leads by example!

Trying to reduce exposure to germs and to people with infections can go a long way in avoiding infections. The easiest and most important thing to do for prevention of infection is good hand washing with soap and water. Antibacterial soaps have not been shown to be much better than regular soap in reducing infections, and any soap is effective—it just must be used! Alcohol-based products and other means of cleansing the hands are also effective in reducing the number of viruses and bacteria on the hands. Routine hand washing is important to general good **hygiene**, but is especially important after contact with someone with an infection (or contact with items the ill person has touched), after contact with animals or pets, after going to the bathroom, before eating, and after any suspected exposures to germs. Infected droplets from anyone with an infection can hide and last for some time on solid objects, so hand washing is key to prevention of transmission to others. Avoiding direct exposure to someone with a significant illness is also common sense, as is staying home from school or work if you yourself have a significant infection which you believe is contagious to others. Children are exposed to a large number of infections in day care environments, church nurseries, schools, and from brothers and sisters, so it is difficult to completely avoid contact with viruses and bacteria. Luckily, development of immunity after routine immunizations, as well as after natural infections by other germs, help strengthen your child's immune system and lead to better overall health.

THE BASICS

Antibacterial soaps have not been shown to be much better than regular soap in reducing infections, and any soap is effective—it just must be used!

Hygiene

Practices such as washing hands, bathing, and brushing teeth which are associated with general cleanliness and ensuring good health.

Amy Lynn's comments:

WASH HANDS!!! Using an anti-bacterial soap regularly with your children and having them wash their hands frequently is a big help. Also, plenty of sleep, healthy foods, and being outside as much as possible.

PART TWO

Are Vaccines Safe?

Are vaccines safe?

Who tests vaccines for safety?
How can they make sure a vaccine is safe?

What are the possible side effects of a vaccine?

More . . .

10. Are vaccines safe?

Just like any medication, no vaccine is 100% safe. The same can be said of the food we eat, the beverages we drink, and the activities in which we participate. There is always going to be some degree of risk. Many people, and not just the drug manufacturers, think that the current vaccines used in the United States are the safest in history.

Vaccines are tested for years prior to licensing for use, and afterwards are monitored very closely for any indications of lack of safety. Problems that arise can, and should, be reported to the national **Vaccine Adverse Event Reporting System (VAERS)**. The VAERS, which is also mentioned in the answers to questions 22 and 23, is a national passive reporting system that accepts reports from the public (doctors, nurses, parents, anyone) on adverse events associated with any vaccine licensed in the United States. Since 1990, more than 123,000 reports have been filed, the majority by vaccine manufacturers. Most reports, approximately 85%, describe fever and other minor reactions as the adverse event. However, the other 15% of reports have described more serious events. Many of these events are found not to relate to the vaccine itself, but all are reviewed. VAERS data reports are checked continuously to pick up previously unknown adverse effects or any increase in adverse events. If a safety concern exists, action can be taken, including discontinuing the vaccine.

When people experience adverse effects of vaccines, it is usually in the form of a mild local reaction at the site of the shot. More severe side effects, including allergic reactions, are rare. However, it is important for a parent to be informed of these reactions. Your doctor should not only discuss the risks of vaccines with you before your child gets each vaccine, but also give you a form called a **Vaccine Information Statement (VIS)**. The VIS is a

Vaccine Adverse Event Reporting System (VAERS)

A national reporting system in the United States that accepts reports from the public (doctors, nurses, parents, anyone) regarding adverse events associated with any vaccine licensed in the United States.

Vaccine Information Statement (VIS)

A form developed by the Center for Disease Control and Prevention (CDC) which provides information on the risks and benefits of individual vaccines.

form developed by the Center for Disease Control and Prevention (CDC) for the purpose of ensuring that every vaccine recipient, or parent/guardian of a child receiving a vaccine, is informed of the risks and benefits of each vaccine. All doctors and health care providers giving vaccines are required to give the patient or their parent/guardian the most current VIS available for each vaccine, give them time to read the VIS, record in the chart the date the VIS was given, and record the publication date of the VIS. While this mandate is meant to emphasize the importance of this written information, the VIS is not meant to replace direct discussions between you and your child's doctor, and all questions and concerns should be discussed before any vaccine is given.

The VIS is not meant to replace direct discussions between you and your child's doctor, and all questions and concerns should be discussed before any vaccine is given.

In any discussion of safety, one has to discuss the issue in terms of benefits and risks. In other words, do the benefits of giving a vaccine to your child outweigh the risk of the vaccine to your child? For most children in the United States, with the currently available vaccines, that answer is yes. Vaccines protect children from many serious diseases. Vaccines work so well that, with the exception of the elderly and some foreign immigrants, people in the United States have not had to experience the fear of many diseases such as polio, congenital rubella, diphtheria, measles, and many others that caused so much serious illness, long-term complications, and death in children. The decision to give your child vaccines is important because it affects not only your child, but your family and the health and safety of the community.

There are many sources of good information, specifically on vaccine safety, benefits of vaccines, and general information to help you decide whether to give vaccines to your child. The appendix in this book contains a list of many books, web sites, and other resources with this information.

Mary Ellen's comments:

I am glad to have this question answered clearly! The resources provided in the appendix are another positive.

11. Who tests vaccines for safety? How can they make sure a vaccine is safe?

Vaccines are like any other prescription drug when it comes to the process of approving it for use in children. Vaccines are given to children only after a long process of review and testing for safety and efficacy. Different groups are then responsible for licensing the vaccine, recommending it for use, and possibly requiring its use.

As discussed in the answer to question 4, vaccines are made only after many years of research by scientists obtaining a good understanding of the virus or bacterium, especially how it causes disease. Then researchers can make a decision about what is the best type of vaccine to use to prevent infection by the germ and/or the disease caused by the germ. This decision is made with careful attention to efficacy and safety.

Vaccines are usually made by first showing that they are safe and effective in experimental animals. Once this is established, the vaccine becomes an **Investigational New Drug** (**IND**) and the company is given an IND license to further study the safety and effectiveness of the vaccine in adults, and eventually in children. These clinical trials usually take many years, giving companies ample time to provide the U.S. **Food and Drug Administration (FDA)** with proof of long-term safety and effectiveness. Much of the early research may be done in university research laboratories or in other private research or pharmaceutical company laboratories,

Investigational New Drug (IND)

An official designation by the United States Food and Drug Administration (FDA) for an experimental vaccine that has not yet been approved for marketing.

Food and Drug Administration (FDA)

The agency which is part of the United States Department of Health and Human Services which is responsible for the safety regulation of many items, including vaccines.

but subsequent studies for licensing are performed by the pharmaceutical companies. In addition to taking many years to complete, these studies are also costly.

Three phases of studies are done prior to licensing a vaccine; they are called Phase I, II, and III. In Phase I studies, a small number of people, usually healthy adults, are given the vaccine to make sure it is safe and determine whether it produces immunity or antibodies in their blood. If results are good, the Phase II study begins, testing the vaccine in a larger number of people, usually the population in which the vaccine will be used. Safety and immune response are again analyzed. Again, if study results look good, Phase III studies are conducted. These are very large clinical trials, studying thousands of people to make sure the vaccine is safe and that it works. All the results from these clinical studies are then submitted to scientists and regulatory personnel at the United States Food and Drug Administration (FDA). It is their responsibility to review how all the studies were done and to make sure the results showed that the vaccine is safe and that it works. The FDA may not approve the vaccine, or they may require additional studies to be done to prove its safety. If it does appear to be a safe and effective vaccine, the FDA can give its approval to license the drug for use.

After this process, the next step is to decide whether the vaccine should be put into general use in the United States. Recommendations are sought from the **Advisory Committee on Immunization Practices** (**ACIP**), which is part of the **Centers for Disease Control and Prevention** (**CDC**). Committees representing other experts who care for children, including the Committee on Infectious Diseases of the **American Academy of Pediatrics** (**AAP**) and the **American Academy of Family Physicians** (**AAFP**), also provide recommendations. These groups again review

Advisory Committee on Immunization Practices (ACIP)

A committee that gives official federal guidance and recommendations on the use of vaccines and the vaccine schedules in the United States.

Centers for Disease Control and Prevention (CDC)

An agency in the United States Department of Health and Social Services which works with local health departments and many other agencies to promote health, as well as prevention and control of diseases, in the United States.

American Academy of Pediatrics (AAP)

An organization of pediatricians who are advocates for children's health.

American Academy of Family Physicians (AAFP)

An organization of family physicians with a mission to promote the health of patients, families, and communities.

ARE VACCINES SAFE?

the data on safety and efficacy and consider the costs and benefits of the vaccine. These groups then make a final recommendation that doctors can follow in deciding who should receive the vaccine. After this, the state legislatures and health departments in each state must make a decision as to whether the vaccine will be required in that state. This decision is based, in part, on economics.

After a vaccine is distributed for use, additional studies occur; these are ongoing for as long as the vaccine is in use. Vaccine safety is continually monitored by the CDC to make sure there are not some rare side effects of a vaccine which were not detected in all the prior safety studies. The CDC does this in several ways. Certain health departments across the nation monitor everyone who gets the vaccine to look for adverse effects. The CDC closely tracks reportable diseases or adverse events reported to any health department to check for the relationship of those diseases or events with the administration of any vaccine. The CDC also reviews information from the VAERS, or Vaccine Adverse Events Reporting System. The VAERS is a reporting system where anyone—doctor, nurse, or parent—who thinks a vaccine caused a significant side effect can file a report. This system is monitored, and reports are reviewed to see if there is any link between the vaccine and the side effects. Lastly, there is a large database called the **Vaccine Safety Datalink (VSD)**, which includes millions of people and follows those who received vaccines to assess any safety concerns.

Vaccine Safety Datalink (VSD)

A project of the CDC and eight large managed care organizations which monitors a large population of patients in the United States to assess vaccine safety.

Unfortunately, no evaluation system can guarantee the safety of a vaccine. Perhaps of greatest concern is that a vaccine might cause or contribute to an adverse effect which is significantly delayed in onset, especially if the adverse effects are subtle. However, use of all the monitoring and reporting systems previously described provide an assessment of short-term and long-term effects of vaccines, and these systems combine to create a thorough and effective system for evaluation of vaccine safety.

12. What are the possible side effects of a vaccine?

Although there are many possible side effects of vaccines, most children either do quite well and experience no adverse effect or have only minor side effects after getting a vaccine. Reactions to vaccines can be categorized as local, systemic, and allergic. The most common are local side effects which involve a reaction at the injection site. Although some children have no evidence of having a shot, there can be some redness, tenderness, and swelling at the place on the skin where the shot was given. This may start a few hours after getting the vaccine and usually lasts from a few hours to a few days. Systemic reactions include any type of vaccine effects that involve the whole body. The most common systemic reactions are mild fever, irritability, fatigue, muscle aches, headache, and loss of appetite. These usually last a maximum of a few days. It is sometimes difficult to determine whether these are due to a vaccine or some other infection, such as a cold or ear infection, unrelated to the vaccine.

Luckily, allergic reactions to vaccines are very uncommon, but they are also the most severe. There is a range of allergic reactions, but the most severe can be life-threatening. This type of reaction usually occurs if the child has an allergy to a part of the vaccine (for example, the child has an allergy to eggs and the vaccine administered has traces of egg protein). The risk of a severe allergic reaction is about one in a million with such an allergy. This reaction can start within minutes or after a couple of hours and may include

The risk of a severe allergic reaction is about one in a million.

hives, problems breathing, wheezing, dizziness, pale skin, and rapid heart rate. Doctor's offices are well-prepared to deal with these reactions. Their occurrence, though rare, makes it important for the parent to always tell your doctor if your child has any known allergies.

Amy Lynn's comments:

The most common side effects we have seen are slight swelling or discomfort around the area of the shot and low-grade fevers.

13. Are there harmful additives or chemicals in vaccines?

The major ingredient in a vaccine is the killed or weakened microorganism, or part of the microorganism, which is included to stimulate the body to build an immune response. But fluids and chemical additives are included in the vaccine preparation to make sure that the vaccine remains safe, sterile, and potent until it is given to your child. Therefore, the final vaccine product can contain a variety of substances including the diluent, adjuvants, stabilizers, antibiotics and preservatives, and other remnants from the vaccine manufacturing process.

The **diluent** is the liquid used to dilute the vaccine to the right dose; this is often water or saline (water with salt). **Adjuvants** are substances added to the vaccine to improve the immune response by making it occur earlier, more potent or longer lasting. Aluminum salts are a common adjuvant. **Stabilizers** are added to help the vaccine stay potent even through changes in temperature, humidity, light, or acidity. Common stabilizers include MSG (monosodium glutamate), albumin (protein), phenols, gelatin, and glycine. Antibiotics can

Diluent

The liquid used to dilute a vaccine to the right dose.

Adjuvants

Substances added to a vaccine to help make the immune response earlier, more potent or longer lasting.

Stabilizers

Substances added to a vaccine to help the vaccine stay potent even with changes in temperature, humidity, light, or acidity. MSG (monosodium glutamate) and albumin (protein) are two examples of stabilizers used in vaccines.

be added during the manufacturing process to prevent other bacteria from contaminating the vaccine cultures. Other **preservatives** are also added to make sure the vaccine stays sterile. One formerly used preservative was **thimerosal**; most vaccines do not use this any longer, as is discussed in a later question in this section.

Some substances might be used during production of the vaccine and then removed from the final product; however, it is sometimes difficult to determine whether trace amounts of these substances are sometimes present in the final vaccine. Things in this category include substances in the cultures of the organism (e.g., egg proteins) and chemicals used to inactivate the organisms (formaldehyde). Some people are concerned with the presence of even trace amounts of some additives, but scientists with expertise in this area believe the amounts of these substances left in vaccines are too small to create any adverse effects.

For further information on what exact chemicals or additives a specific vaccine contains, your doctor or pharmacist can give you a copy of the vaccine package insert. This document lists all of the ingredients in the vaccine and presents information about any known adverse reactions. The same information can also be accessed via internet websites. The Johns Hopkins Institute for Vaccine Safety has created a website with valuable information, including a table which lists all the components of the common vaccines. The information is organized to allow searching all vaccines for a specific inactive substance or by active component, or separately to examine all the components of a specific vaccine. The link to this table is *http://www.vaccinesafety.edu/components.htm*.

Preservatives

Substances added to a vaccine to help the vaccine remain sterile.

Thimerosal

A vaccine preservative which contains ethylmercury.

ARE VACCINES SAFE?

14. How do you know if your child is allergic to a vaccine?

The vaccine information statement given to you before your child gets a vaccine should provide information about important components of the vaccine to which your child might be allergic. If you know your child is allergic or has a history of having any serious reaction to any of the substances in the vaccine, you should discuss this with your doctor before the vaccine is given. Not infrequently, children have had a rash or other minor reaction with certain foods, drugs, or with a prior vaccine. This should be discussed with the physician before your child gets the vaccine. Severe allergic reactions, or hypersensitivity reactions, often start within minutes to a few hours after exposure to the substance, and the signs and symptoms may include hives, problems breathing, wheezing, dizziness, pale appearance, and rapid heart rate. Any child who has this type of reaction to a vaccine should not receive another dose of that vaccine. Your child's doctor may consult a specialist in pediatric allergy if there is any question about the type of reaction and whether subsequent vaccines should be given.

Amy Lynn's comments:
Your pediatrician should give you a specific list of things to watch for in regards to the specific vaccine, but any out of the ordinary behavior such as breathing difficulty, high fever, rash, etc. should be noted and reported immediately.

15. Do vaccines cause autism?

Autism is a term often used to refer to a group of developmental disorders that affect the brain. Autism is one of five related developmental and neurological disorders called **autism spectrum disorders (ASDs)**. Autism,

Autism

A term often used to refer to a group of developmental disorders that affect the brain. (*See* Autism spectrum disorders).

Autism spectrum disorders (ASDs)

A group of five related developmental and neurological disorders that affect the brain.

pervasive developmental disorder—not otherwise specified (PDD-NOS), and Asperger's Syndrome are three disorders in this group. Children with ASDs have a range of disabilities, but often have difficulty in their ability to communicate, form relationships with others, and respond to their environment. People with autism may also show significant repetition in certain behaviors and interests and have rigid patterns of thought. While some children with autism have severe cognitive and language delays, and may have little to no speech, others have normal intelligence and speech and are able to function well.

Early signs of autism, especially with differences in social skills and language, can sometimes be detected during infancy. An infant with autism may avoid eye contact, appear deaf, and seem to stop developing language and social skills. However, because activities like sitting, crawling and walking are often not delayed, these differences often go unnoticed. The diagnosis is often apparent by age three, but due to the variation in severity and presentation, it can be evident earlier, or sometimes much later.

There is a strong genetic basis for autism, and having one child in the family with this diagnosis increases the likelihood of having other children with autism. The causes of autism remain unclear, but evidence exists that a variety of factors are associated with forms of autism, including genetic, metabolic, infectious, neurological, and environmental factors, including exposure to specific foods, medications, or toxins. Unfortunately the incidence of autism in the United States is rising, and currently the estimate is that autism occurs in 1 in 150 children. This increase is probably due to multiple reasons, including a change in the definition of ASD, increase in doctors' recognition and diagnosis of ASD, and possibly a true increase in ASD. There is no definitive cure and ASDs are lifelong conditions. However, children can improve developmentally and learn new skills; and some children can improve to the point they no longer meet criteria for a diagnosis of ASD.

Recognition of the symptoms of autism and diagnosis of the disorder most often occur in the first two to three years of life. Since children receive immunizations during this time period, there has been concern that a vaccine or vaccine component causes autism. Most concerns have been associated with the presence of a mercury compound, thimerosal, in vaccines and with the combined measles, mumps, and rubella (MMR) vaccine. The issue of thimerosal is discussed in question 16 and the question of a link between the MMR vaccine and autism is discussed here.

One study which led to increased interest in the possible link between the MMR vaccine and autism involved an analysis of data from children in California. The data showed an increase in the number of children diagnosed with autism since children started receiving the MMR vaccine. Other scientists who reviewed the data disagreed with the suggestion that the MMR vaccine in any way caused autism. These scientists pointed out that the number of autism cases was known to rise during the time period due to improved diagnosis, changes in the definition of autism which increased the number of cases, and simply increase in the population of children in California.

Two studies from England, published in 1998 and 2002, presented data on a group of children with autism and bowel disease. A small group of children with autism was examined for evidence of measles virus in the bowel.

Results of the study showed some evidence of the virus in a high percentage of children with autism, but in only a few children who did not have autism. These scientists proposed that autism was caused by a process involving the vaccine, bowel inflammation, and subsequent damage to the brain. Other scientists have also evaluated this data, and have found errors, some minor and some more significant, which bring into question the conclusions of the study. Nevertheless, studies such as this led to concern that the vaccine may have some relationship with autism.

In early 2008, one family in the United States was awarded compensation through the federal Vaccine Injury Compensation Program after their child developed signs of autism. Although full details of this child's medical history have not yet been made public, the child is reported to have an underlying disease called a **mitochondrial disorder**, one in a group of diseases which can affect the brain and can be associated with various neurologic symptoms which become more severe as the child ages. The main issue discussed in this case was whether the administration of vaccines to this child may have aggravated her underlying disease and resulted in a brain disorder with the features of autism. The award of compensation for this family has led to further controversy and significant discussions about whether the use of some vaccines such as the MMR can adversely affect children, specifically those with certain underlying genetic diseases, by either causing autism or providing the stimulus which brings out the symptoms of autism. After the announcement of this settlement, several agencies involved with vaccine safety have repeated their assertion that there is no evidence that the MMR or other vaccines cause autism.

Mitochondrial disorder

A specific type of disease which can affect the brain and can be associated with various neurologic symptoms which become more severe as the child ages.

Epidemiologic studies have been conducted in several European countries as well as in the United States, to investigate whether any association could be detected between the MMR vaccine and the development of autism. Results from Sweden, Denmark, England, and the United States have failed to detect any link between the vaccine and autism. Other types of research have examined "home videos" of infants who were later diagnosed with autism. These studies showed that some infants exhibit detectable evidence of autism at an age prior to receiving the MMR vaccine. Research is ongoing to try to better understand the causes of autism. To date, genetics and events occurring during pregnancy seem to be highly implicated as risk factors for autism. The current consensus among groups of experts, including the American Academy of Pediatrics and the **Institute of Medicine**, is still that data do not support a causal relationship or link between vaccines, specifically the MMR vaccine, and the development of autism.

To date, genetics and events occurring during pregnancy seem to be highly implicated as risk factors for autism.

Institute of Medicine

A non-governmental agency which provides health information to policy-makers, healthcare professionals, and the general public.

16. Do vaccines still have thimerosal (mercury) in them and can that make children ill?

It has long been known that exposure to mercury can be dangerous and can affect the brain and nervous system. Because many vaccines used to contain (and a small number still contain) the additive thimerosal, a mercury-containing compound, there has been concern that the mercury from vaccines could harm a young infant. Since high concentrations of mercury affect the brain, the possibility that this additive causes autism has been proposed.

Mercury is an element present in the earth's crust, soil, water, and air. It occurs in three different forms, elemental, inorganic, and organic mercury. Elemental mercury is the form of mercury found in older glass thermometers. Organic mercury is the form in some environmental and food sources and is important because it is absorbed and gets across the bloodstream fairly well. Because mercury is found throughout the environment, it is also found in our food and water. For example, there has been recent concern about the high mercury levels in certain types of fish. It is even present in trace amounts in infant formula (from water), as well as in breast milk. The mercury in breast milk, which comes from sources such as amalgam fillings in teeth and fish in the mother's diet, has been shown to be safe for the infant.

High concentrations of mercury in the body are known to affect both the brain and nervous system. Mercury's effects on the brain were described in the character with "mad hatter syndrome" in Lewis Carroll's *Alice in Wonderland*. Hat makers in the 19th century used mercury in part of the hat-making process, and the high exposures led to various neurologic symptoms. Acute mercury poisoning has occurred several times in history, including in Iraq in the 1970s due to mercury-contaminated grain, and in Japan during the 1950s due to consumption of fish with high levels of methylmercury, a form of organic mercury. Effects were seen in adults, children, and infants born to women with high exposures during pregnancy. Epidemiologic studies on these affected children showed various neurologic deficits and more subtle developmental delays, but no increased frequency of autism.

Thimerosal is a compound which contains ethylmercury. **Ethylmercury** is an organic mercury similar to **methylmercury**, but it is excreted faster from the body and, in a small study, was found to be less toxic. Since

Ethylmercury

A type of organic compound which contains mercury.

Methylmercury

One type of organic compound which contains mercury.

Food and Drug Administration Modernization Act

Legislation passed by the United States Congress which was geared to streamline the process of bringing safe and effective drugs, medical devices, and other therapies to the United States market.

The consensus from the scientific community is that there is no evidence that thimerosal caused any illness in children, including autism or any other type of neurologic damage. Additional studies have shown that autism occurs at the same rate in children who received vaccines with thimerosal and those who did not.

the 1930s, thimerosal has been used as a preservative in vaccines because it is effective in preventing contamination of vaccines by bacteria and yeast. As the risks of mercury in the environment became more apparent, the use of mercury-containing additives began to be questioned. There was specific concern that autism, a group of developmental disorders that affect the brain (see question 15), might be caused by thimerosal. In 1997, an amendment to the **Food and Drug Administration Modernization Act** started the process to remove thimerosal from vaccines. In 1999, vaccine manufacturers were told to eliminate or reduce the use of thimerosal as a precaution. Now, thimerosal is no longer used as a preservative in almost all vaccines. Some types of influenza vaccine, multi-dose vials of a meningococcal vaccine (Menomune), and some preparations of vaccines with the tetanus toxoid still have trace amounts of thimerosal (concentrations of 0.01%). You can ask your child's doctor if a specific vaccine has any trace of thimerosal, review the vaccine information given to you, or access the information on many vaccine safety websites. The Johns Hopkins Institute for Vaccine Safety keeps an updated table on the content of thimerosal in vaccines. The link to this table is *http://www.vaccinesafety.edu/thi-table.htm.*

The consensus from the scientific community is that there is no evidence that thimerosal caused any illness in children, including autism or any other type of neurologic damage. Additional studies have shown that autism occurs at the same rate in children who received vaccines with thimerosal and those who did not. In Denmark, thimerosal was discontinued in 1991, and autism cases have continued to increase despite discontinuation of this preservative. In January of 2008, an epidemiologic study of autism in children in California from 1995 to

2007 was published. This study, as well as others, has shown that despite the decreased exposure to thimerosal, frequency of autism has continued to rise. Therefore, current data give no indication that the use of thimerosal was linked with autism. Continuing epidemiologic data is being gathered and vaccine-associated events are being carefully followed to monitor vaccine safety. Research to further clarify causes of autism also continues.

17. Can vaccines cause SIDS (sudden infant death syndrome)?

A popular television documentary aired a story about one infant who died of **sudden infant death syndrome (SIDS)** 16 hours after receiving her hepatitis B vaccine. Before introduction of this vaccine, about 5,000 children died with SIDS every year. There has been a dramatic decrease in the number of SIDS deaths, with current estimates being approximately 1,600 per year. This significant decrease is attributed primarily to the national "Back to Sleep" program for infants. Statistically, with this many cases of SIDS, it would be expected that about 50 infants would die of SIDS within 24 hours of receiving a vaccine. The incidence of SIDS is the same in infants who receive vaccines and those who do not. Therefore, there is no evidence that the hepatitis B vaccine, or any vaccine, contributes to the number of infants dying of SIDS.

18. Can vaccines cause MS (multiple sclerosis) or other autoimmune diseases?

Because vaccines stimulate the immune system during the process of creating a protective immune response, there has long been interest as to whether vaccines can cause or exacerbate the symptoms of specific autoimmune diseases.

Sudden infant death syndrome (SIDS)

A term used to denote the sudden and unexplained death of an apparently healthy infant aged one month to one year.

The incidence of SIDS is the same in infants who receive vaccines and those who do not. Therefore, there is no evidence that the hepatitis B vaccine, or any vaccine, contributes to the number of infants dying of SIDS.

Multiple sclerosis (MS)

A chronic, progressive disease that involves the brain, spinal cord, and other parts of the central nervous system.

Multiple sclerosis (MS) is a chronic, progressive disease that involves the brain, spinal cord, and other parts of the central nervous system. It is called an autoimmune disease because the body's own immune system is involved with the disease process by targeting the body's own cells, tissues and organs. Several scientific studies have examined whether certain vaccines (including hepatitis B, tetanus, or influenza vaccine) were associated with the risk of MS or exacerbation of symptoms in MS patients. Results of the studies showed that the vaccines studied did not cause or exacerbate the symptoms of MS.

Other diseases with an immune basis have been studied to examine links with a vaccine. No link to diabetes has been found with any vaccine. Asthma is more of an allergic disease although with immune-mediated processes. Vaccines have not been found to be associated with asthma.

No link to diabetes has been found with any vaccine. Asthma is more of an allergic disease although with immune-mediated processes. Vaccines have not been found to be associated with asthma.

19. Are there some children who should not get vaccines?

Most children can receive all recommended vaccines, but there are some important exceptions. If your child has had a previous severe reaction to a vaccine, such as breathing problems, low blood pressure, or severe hives, the vaccine should not be given. Likewise, if your child has a severe allergy to a known component of a vaccine (e.g., an egg allergy for MMR vaccine), that vaccine should not be given. Some children have a weakened immune system due to a known immune deficiency, cancer, or another underlying disease. Depending on the degree of immune suppression, the live, attenuated virus vaccines (e.g., measles, mumps, rubella, rotavirus, and varicella) may be contraindicated. Medications such as high dose steroids may also weaken the immune system to the point that vaccines should be delayed. If your child has been taking high dose steroids (high dose is considered to be 2 milligrams (mg) per kilogram or more of prednisone per day), the live attenuated virus vaccines should be delayed. At the time of vaccine administration, your care provider should review contraindications for each vaccine as well as review your child's current health to insure that vaccine administration should proceed.

20. My daughter might be pregnant. Do any vaccines harm the fetus?

It is important for all women of child-bearing age to stay up-to-date on their immunizations, not only for their own protection but to provide the best protection for their infants. Antibodies which the mother has will be transferred to her infant during the last trimester of pregnancy, helping to protect the infant from many different infections during the first few months of life. Specific vaccines for which a pregnant woman is advised to be up-to-date include influenza, hepatitis B, tetanus, and pneumococcus, if needed. However, the use of live virus vaccines during pregnancy should be avoided due to the possibility, even though it is remote, that the fetus might be affected. Therefore, the MMR (measles, mumps, and rubella) and the varicella vaccine are currently not recommended during pregnancy. Also, the live influenza vaccine is not advised for a pregnant woman, but the inactivated influenza vaccine is recommended for use during pregnancy.

21. Can others catch an infection after being with a recently immunized person?

Killed vaccines, subunit vaccines, and toxoid vaccines do not transmit infections. A vaccine-associated infection acquired after the receipt of a live, weakened virus vaccine would be the only scenario which could, in theory, lead to an infection being transmitted to another individual. Historically, the oral polio vaccine (a live virus vaccine, no longer used in the United States) was thought to be contagious enough and dangerous enough to someone with a weakened immune system that it was not recommended for use in certain situations. The MMR (measles, mumps, and rubella vaccine), varicella vaccine, and the rotavirus vaccine are the only live, attenuated vaccines in the routine immunization schedule for children. Although children receiving these viruses can have small amounts of the weakened virus detected in their mouths or stools for a couple of weeks after immunization, the virus is present in such a weakened form and in such little amounts that the risk for any family members is thought to be minimal, even if they have an extremely weakened immune system. Therefore, these vaccines are not contraindicated to be given to children living in the same household. As noted, all other routine vaccines are either killed or in a form that they cannot produce an active infection in either the vaccine recipient or in anyone in contact with them.

Most children do not have any reactions with a vaccine, and when they occur most of them are minor.

22. What do I do if my child has a reaction to a vaccine?

Most children do not have any reactions with a vaccine, and when they occur most of them are minor. The most common reactions are local reactions (tenderness, redness, warmth at the site of the shot) or mild systemic reactions such as mild fever or irritability. Your doctor should discuss and give instructions as to what to do for reactions when the vaccines are given (if not, please ask!). If you think your child has a fever, you should check their temperature with a thermometer. For mild fever, doctors often recommend things like giving the child plenty of fluids, use of light (not heavy) clothing, giving the appropriate dose of a medicine such as acetaminophen or ibuprofen (not aspirin), giving your child a sponge-bath in lukewarm water, and keeping close watch of the temperature (recheck in an hour). Your doctor may give you guidelines on when to call the doctor (i.e. the degree of fever). Use of a cool washcloth at the site of the local reaction can help to soothe the skin. The above-noted medications may also be advised to help soothe the local reaction, as well as for some minor irritability. If fever, irritability, or the local reaction gets worse or persists beyond 24–48 hours, you should at least contact your doctor for further advice. If, at any time, you are concerned about the reaction, or if your child ever has any reaction to a vaccine which you think is serious, you should contact your doctor or take your child to a doctor immediately. You should definitely call if the fever/temperature is above the level that you were told to call, if your child looks pale or limp and shows decreased activity, if he has body jerking or shaking, or if he has persistent crying or a high-pitched cry lasting more than three hours.

If your child has a severe or important reaction to a vaccine, or if your child has any medical problem you think might be associated with or caused by a vaccine, it should be reported. The national VAERS (Vaccine Adverse Event Reporting System) collects any and all reports of suspected vaccine injuries. Although the doctor usually completes this form and sends it to the program, any parent or individual can file a report. You can get more information by calling the VAERS toll-free at 1-800-822-7967 or by visiting their website at *www.vaers.hhs.gov*. Not all reactions reported to VAERS are caused by the vaccine, and they may be unrelated; however, all reports contribute useful information to make sure vaccines are safe, and any concern of a significant reaction should be reported.

Amy Lynn's comments:

Immediately contact your pediatrician—if it is severe (such as trouble breathing) you should take your child to an emergency room and take the information about the vaccine they received.

23. What is the National Childhood Vaccine Injury Act?

National Childhood Vaccine Injury Act (NCVIA)

Legislation passed in 1986 to help protect vaccine makers from the financial liability involved with lawsuits arising from vaccine injury.

The main purpose of the **National Childhood Vaccine Injury Act (NCVIA)** of 1986 was to help protect vaccine makers from the financial liability involved with lawsuits involving vaccine injury. The legislation was designed to help make the vaccine market stable and to help provide cost-effective arbitration for vaccine injury claims. Under the NCVIA, the National Vaccine Injury Compensation Program (NVICP) was created to provide a claim system procedure in the United States Court of Federal Claims system for compensating vaccine-related injuries or death. If your child were ever to suffer a serious injury associated with receipt of a vaccine, this program may provide compensation to you to help with the care of your child. Information about this program can be obtained by calling their toll-free number at 1-800-338-2382 or looking at their website *www.hrsa.gov/vaccinecompensation*. Legal consultation to discuss the injury and for you to fully understand your, and your child's, rights and options is encouraged.

The NCVIA also created several other new requirements relating to various aspects of vaccine safety. It was
this Act which required all doctors and other health care
providers to report adverse effects which were noted after
vaccination to the Vaccine Adverse Event Reporting
System (VAERS) described in the answers to previous questions. It also established a committee from the
Institute of Medicine (IOM) to review current literature
and reports on all adverse effects associated with immunization, whether or not there was thought to be a direct
link of the event to the vaccine. The National Vaccine
Program Office (NVPO) was created to coordinate all
immunization-related activities among various government agencies including the Center for Disease Control
and Prevention (CDC), the Food and Drug Association
(FDA), the National Institute of Health (NIH), and
other agencies. In addition, the NCVIA required all
doctors and health care providers who administer any
of the common vaccines to give Vaccine Information
Statements (VIS) to the person getting the vaccine or
to their parent or guardian. As discussed previously, the
VIS is the document produced by the CDC which is
given to you each time your child receives a vaccine. The
VIS contains a brief description of the disease and out-
lines the benefits and risks of the vaccine. It is designed
to make sure the person receiving the vaccine or their
parent or guardian is well informed about the vaccine.
The mandates for use of the VIS, as well as implementation of other NCVIA requirements, have helped to
improve and increase awareness of vaccine safety issues
in the United States.

24. My doctor asked if I would let my child be in a vaccine study. How do I decide?

Participation in clinical studies for vaccines, as well as for other medicines or therapies, is an important part of the process to make available new and improved medicines and vaccines. Many doctors are involved with clinical studies of various types, including studies on new or improved vaccines. While participation in the studies is quite important, you need to be well-informed before you allow your child to participate. Your doctor should give you materials to read and should discuss the clinical study with you. You should have a full understanding of all aspects of the vaccine and the clinical study. Usually you will be asked to sign an official consent form giving your permission for your child to participate. If your child is old enough, sometimes your child is also given a consent form. All of your, and your child's, questions about the study should be well discussed and answered to your satisfaction prior to signing the forms and before participation in the study.

Examples of questions you should ask, or have answered, regarding a clinical study are as follows:

- What is the name of this study?
- Who is the principal investigator (person running the study)?
- What is the purpose of this study?
- Are there any reasons my child should not be in the study?
- How many children will take part in this study?
- How long will my child's part in the study last?
- What will happen if my child takes part in the study?

- What are the possible benefits from being in the study?
- What are the possible risks or discomforts involved with being in this study?
- If my child is not in the study, what other treatment options (or vaccine options) does my child have?
- What if we learn about new findings or information during the study?
- How will my child's privacy be protected?
- What will happen if my child is injured by this research?
- What if my child wants to stop before our part in the study is complete?
- Will I or my child receive anything for being in this study?
- Will it cost anything to be in this study?
- Who is sponsoring this study?
- What if I or my child has questions about the rights of my child as a research subject?

Often, the answers to these questions are outlined in the official consent to participate in the study. Again, both you and your child should have all questions answered before consenting to participate. There are many rewards, and often opportunities, in participating in a clinical research study, but benefits and risks must always be considered.

PART THREE

Giving Vaccines to Children

Do I have to give my children vaccines?

What are the risks of not using vaccines for my child?

Isn't a baby protected if the pregnant mother was up-to-date with her vaccines?

More . . .

25. Do I have to give my children vaccines?

The decision to give or not to give vaccines to a child is the decision of the parent or official guardian.

The decision to give or not to give vaccines to a child is the decision of the parent or official guardian. The decision to immunize your child, and decisions pertaining to any medical care for your child, should be made in consideration of your child's best interest. Although medical decision-making, including decisions on the use of vaccines, should be shared between the health care provider and the parents, permission of the parents must be granted before your child receives a medical intervention, and this includes a vaccine. Parents are free to make choices regarding immunizations, or any medical care, unless those choices place your child at significant risk of severe harm.

Whether refusal of immunization places your child at risk of serious harm depends upon the probability of contracting the disease if unimmunized and the morbidity and mortality associated with infection. The role of the health care provider should be to provide parents with the risk and benefit information needed to make an informed decision and to correct misinformation or misinterpretations. It is rare that the decision of the parents regarding immunizations is thought to be of sufficient risk of harm for the child that the health care professional is obliged to involve state agencies to intervene and have the situation further investigated. One example sometimes quoted is if the child had a contaminated cut or wound which was a significant risk for getting tetanus, and the parent refused to let the child have the tetanus vaccine or antibody. The decision would have to be made whether the parent's decision should be challenged. Other situations may arise where others are placed at risk of significant harm by a child's lack of immunization. In times of epidemic disease, when an effective and safe vaccine can interrupt the epidemic and protect people who have not had the infection, overriding a vaccine refusal may be considered. Regardless, it is the parent's right, and their responsibility, to be fully informed of the risks and benefits of vaccines for children in order to make the best decision for their child.

26. What are the risks of not using vaccines for my child?

For many children who do not receive vaccines, there are no adverse consequences. They may never be exposed to the diseases which vaccines prevent, and therefore may not get the illness. They may be exposed to some of the vaccine-preventable diseases and not have a severe illness. However, for many diseases, if an unvaccinated child is exposed to someone with the disease, there is a good chance they will get the disease. The result of all the infections described in this book are quite varied, and range from no obvious symptoms or disease, to illnesses which are brief and minor, to more severe illnesses which may have severe complications and even death. In addition, there can be severe public health consequences of outbreaks of many types of infections. Infants too young to be immunized, other children and adults who lack immunity, and people with weak immune systems may also get the disease and suffer bad outcomes. Finally, as vaccines are mandated for use in certain settings, including daycares and schools, you will need to determine and understand the consequences, if any, of not giving vaccines to your children.

27. Isn't a baby protected if the pregnant mother was up-to-date with her vaccines?

During pregnancy, and especially in the last trimester of pregnancy, many of the antibodies the mother has in her body start to be transferred to the fetus. Therefore, a newborn infant has some of the mother's antibodies, and these antibodies provide protection to the infant against some infectious agents. In addition, if the mother breastfeeds the baby, additional protection is provided. Breast milk contains antibodies and other immune substances from the mother which have been shown to help provide protection against a variety of germs. Breastfed infants have fewer episodes of ear infections, diarrhea, pneumonia, and other types of bacterial and viral infections compared to infants who are not breast fed.

Use of routine immunizations in early infancy adds to the protection given by the mother and helps the baby stay healthy.

Unfortunately, this protection given by the mother lasts for only a limited period of time, and the infant must start developing his or her own immunity. Immunity against some common childhood diseases, for example pertussis (whooping cough), is not transferred to the infant sufficiently to prevent infection. The vaccines recommended for young infants help build up protection against many of the important and serious infections to which young babies are so susceptible. Use of routine immunizations in early infancy adds to the protection given by the mother and helps the baby stay healthy.

28. Can't I wait until my child is ready to go to school to start vaccines?

Infants and young children are the most vulnerable to infection from common diseases. In addition, many diseases cause a much more severe illness in infants compared with older children and adults. Although many exposures to infections occur in daycares and schools, exposures also frequently occur from brief encounters in stores, doctors' offices, neighbors' homes, and especially from brothers and sisters and parents themselves. International travel is also common today, and chance encounters with individuals who have traveled abroad for business, vacation, mission work, and other activities is not uncommon, raising the risk of infections which are seen at low levels in the United States, but occur much more frequently abroad. One must also remember that transmission of infection can often occur from an individual who appears healthy because they may have an asymptomatic infection or be in the early stages of infection. For all these reasons, it is best to begin the immunization schedule as recommended and not wait.

Amy Lynn's comments:
The vaccines required for children to enter public schools require a series that ideally start at birth—if you tried to "catch up" before starting school, it would not be beneficial to the child, not to mention painful if they got all of them in a rapid sequence.

29. Do you get better protection from catching the disease than by getting the vaccine?

In many cases, the actual infection provides better and longer acting immunity to that disease compared with getting immunity from a vaccine. Natural infection activates all parts of the immune system to optimize your body's response and memory cells to provide long lasting protection. However, there are exceptions to this general principle. For many types of diseases, there are multiple types of the infecting germ. Unfortunately, infection with one type of the bacterium or virus may not provide protection from future infection with other types. Also, organisms like the influenza virus may change every year; therefore, even getting the "flu" one year may not protect you from getting the flu in other years. Some infections do not give the best protection, dependent upon how old you are when you get the infection. Most importantly, getting protection from a disease with a vaccine avoids having to get the disease, and dealing with all the illness and complications of that disease. Therefore, vaccines are preferred to natural infection for many types of infections.

30. Are there homeopathic alternatives to vaccines?

A variety of treatments may be recommended by practitioners of alternative medicine for treatment of illnesses or prevention and health promotion. While some practitioners do advise the use of vaccines, others may recommend other types of therapy. Prior to the vaccine era, homeopathic medicine was used to treat or prevent many diseases. **Nosodes**, used by some practitioners of homeopathy, are a class of remedies prepared from dilutions of material obtained from a person with a specific disease. There are homeopathic kits available from some providers for disease prevention. Although there is historical literature regarding the efficacy of some of these preparations, there is a general lack of scientific data regarding the immunologic effects, safety and efficacy of many of these preparations. Specifically, these preparations have not been shown to yield or create a specific immune response which has long term protection against a specific disease.

Nosodes

A class of remedies used by some practitioners of homeopathy.

The benefits of many alternative therapies, including herbal therapies, are gaining interest and being investigated. It is important to always keep your doctor informed of all medications of any type you are giving to your child, including vitamins, herbs, and other therapies, because occasionally there can be adverse reactions with other medications or age-specific toxicity with certain supplements. At this time, however, most doctors will likely not prescribe or advise the use of homeopathic alternatives to vaccines.

All healthcare providers recognize the benefits and impact of good nutrition and lifestyle on the immune system and overall health. Discussion of your child's nutrition and aspects of their lifestyle should be part of every routine visit with your child's health care provider.

31. Should a sick child get a vaccine?

Your doctor can help make the decision, but in general a child with a mild illness such as a cold, ear infection, mild fever, skin infection, or mild diarrhea can still receive routine vaccines at the time of this illness. Children with mild illnesses still have a good response to vaccines, and this response is comparable to the vaccine response in children who have no symptoms at the time they receive vaccines. Also, studies have shown that there is no increased risk of vaccine-associated side effects in children who have a mild illness at the time they get a vaccine. If there are signs of more severe illness, the immunization should be delayed because some symptoms related to the illness may be misinterpreted as being a reaction to the vaccine. If vaccines are delayed, they should be given as soon as your doctor is satisfied your child is well enough to proceed.

32. Can my child get vaccines without getting shots?

Most vaccines are given by shots, either under the skin or into the muscle. This allows for the body to quickly recognize the vaccine proteins and make antibody in the bloodstream and begin the process of creating immunity. Only a few vaccines can be taken by mouth. These include the vaccines against rotavirus and the no-longer-used oral polio. These viruses usually reproduce in the intestines, so this method of immunization was preferred (see discussion of poliovirus to see why the decision was made to switch to the vaccine given in a shot). The newest influenza vaccine is sprayed into the nose and provides a good immune response when given by this route. Other types of vaccines do not work well when given by mouth or in the nose. Much research is being done to find new ways of giving vaccines, including the placement of a unique type of patch containing vaccine on the skin of the arm. But for now, unfortunately, most vaccines are still given in a shot.

Amy Lynn's comments:

There is an influenza vaccine that is a nasal spray called "Flu Mist" that my older children prefer instead of the shot. There are some higher risks associated with it, especially if you have other younger children in the home, but my older kids love it.

33. Are there risks of getting so many shots or vaccines at the same time?

After birth, an infant is exposed to multitudes of different bacteria. These are normal bacteria which live in and on all people. The infant's immune system starts to process all the new **antigens** and begins making immune responses to many of these microorganisms. The vaccines which a child receives are only a small part of this stimulus to the immune system. Although the number of vaccines has increased through the years, the number of proteins in the vaccines (which act in stimulating the immune system) has actually decreased due to changes in some vaccines. There is no evidence that the current vaccines "overload" your child's immune system; giving this number of vaccines has been shown to be safe and effective with no increase in side effects.

Concern has also been raised by some as to whether the use of so many vaccines weakens the immune system and thereby makes your child more susceptible to infections. Research studies have actually shown that the reverse is true. Immunized children seem to have fewer infections from vaccine-related and non-vaccine related pathogens, compared with unimmunized children. Therefore, instead of weakening the immune system, vaccine administration appears to benefit a child's immune system and provides your child broader protection against infection.

34. Can you give all vaccines in one shot?

There are already several preparations of vaccines which can be combined in a single shot. These are named combination vaccines. Some combination vaccines have been in use for some time (e.g., MMR for measles, mumps, and rubella), while others are relatively new, and there are some currently in development (please refer to **Table 2**). Giving all needed vaccines in one shot would, of course, be desirable. Unfortunately, some vaccine preparations should not be mixed in the same syringe because of reactions between the two vaccines. Before a new combination

Antigens

Any substances foreign to the body that stimulate an immune response.

GIVING VACCINES TO CHILDREN

Immunized children seem to have fewer infections from both vaccine-related and non-vaccine related pathogens, compared with unimmunized children.

vaccine can be approved, it must be proven that each vaccine still works as well in the combination as in the separate vaccines. There will likely be more combination vaccines available in the future, and your doctor can discuss what options are available when they are given.

35. Why are some vaccines "single-shot" and some "multiple-shot"? What is a "booster" vaccine?

The goal of giving vaccines is to give your child a maximum level of protection that lasts for as long a time as possible. The many vaccines that are given vary in regards to how many doses it takes to provide that optimum protection. For some vaccines, the first dose "primes"

Table 2 Combination Vaccines Licensed for Use in the United States, 2008

Vaccine Components	Designation/Abbreviation	Brand Name(s)
Diphtheria, Tetanus, Pertussis	DTaP	Daptacel, Infanrix, Tripedia
Diphtheria, Tetanus	Td	Decavac
Diphtheria, Tetanus	DT	(generic)
Diphtheria, Tetanus, Pertussis	Tdap	Boostrix, Adacel
Diphtheria, Tetanus, Pertussis, Polio, Hepatitis B	DTaP / IPV / HepB	Pediarix
Diphtheria, Tetanus, Pertussis, *Haemophilus influenzae* type b	DTaP / Hib	TriHIBit
Hepatitis A, Hepatitis B	HepA / HepB	Twinrix
Hepatitis B, *Haemophilus influenzae* type b	HepB / Hib	Comvax
Measles, Mumps, Rubella	MMR	M-M-R II
Measles, Mumps, Rubella, Varicella	MMRV	ProQuad

the immune system but does not really give protection against the disease—or it does so only in a lower percentage of people. But a subsequent dose or doses gives most people good protection. Some vaccines give almost everyone some protection, but it is not at the highest level, and the additional doses are geared to optimize everyone's level of protection. And, in some vaccines, the level of protection after the first dose is very good but it does not last long, and the additional doses are given to make the protection last longer. Scientists review these characteristics of vaccines and devise the best schedule with recommended number and timing of shots.

Lastly, there is a different situation for certain types of vaccines. Protection against infection by some germs may not last due to the viruses or bacteria changing from year to year. Influenza is an example of such a virus. As described in questions 62–64, this is one reason why people need an influenza vaccine every year to increase the chances of being protected from influenza.

36. The shots hurt! Isn't there something to make them less painful?

The process of giving shots to a child is often dreaded by the child, by the parent—and sometimes even by the health care provider! Although the actual discomfort involved with the stick of the needle is often minor, the child's fear of the process is often significant. There are some simple things that the parent or health care provider can do which may help avoid some of the fear or discomfort associated with shots. Some of these ideas are best suited for certain age groups of children, and the ideas can be divided into things done before, during, and after the actual procedure of giving the shot.

The goal of giving vaccines is to give your child a maximum level of protection that lasts for as long a time as possible. The many vaccines that are given vary in regards to how many doses it takes to provide that optimum protection.

Older children benefit from being told what is going to occur and the reason for the procedure—that the shot or immunization is to help keep them healthy. Teenagers should learn to participate in their own medical care, and should be encouraged to learn and read about immunizations and the diseases they prevent. School-aged children benefit from verbal reassurance from the parent that, although the shots may sting, the pain usually lasts only for a few seconds. Younger children can be told it is OK to cry, but encourage your child to be brave. Infants can be calmed before the procedure by cuddling and keeping a favorite toy or blanket nearby.

The parent being calm throughout the process goes a long way to help your child because your child will be more anxious if you appear anxious. Distraction at the time the child receives the shot is helpful. During shots, infants may be calmed by touching and talking softly while making eye contact. Breastfeeding or bottle feeding may also provide some ease from the discomfort. Older children are helped by distractions such as talking, singing, and play activities (e.g., hand puppet or toy). Having the child "blow away the pain" by blowing on an object during the shot also provides a distraction. Some providers have had the child blow on a small amount of alcohol placed on the same arm the shot is being given, because the cold sensation may relieve some of the discomfort from the shot. The use of a topical anesthetic applied at the site where the child will receive the shot is not common practice for children's immunizations, but it can be considered for children with significant problems receiving shots. A product called **EMLA cream** can be applied with a patch, but needs to be applied for a long duration (e.g., one hour) prior to the procedure if it is to be effective. A topical **anesthetic** will help in lessening the sensation of pain at the skin, but will not ease the discomfort from intramuscular shots, and therefore may not be very beneficial.

EMLA Cream

A type of topical anesthetic which is commonly used to numb the skin prior to certain medical procedures.

Anesthetic

A drug or substance which can produce decreased sensation or awareness. A topical anesthetic is applied to the skin to numb an area of skin prior to a procedure.

After your child receives shots, appropriate praise and comforting should be given. Some health care providers give prizes such as "stickers" after immunizations. A fun activity planned for after the doctor's visit, such as a special trip to the playground or park, helps to ease the overall process. Further suggestions may be given by the health care provider giving the vaccines—ask them for further advice.

Abby's comments:

I remember the shots I've received as a teenager. I find not looking at the needle to be helpful since seeing the needle can inspire fear. I do feel pain for a few seconds when I'm pricked with a needle, but it is nothing a sparkly Band-Aid and lollipop can't fix. I think teenagers should still get the sparkly Band-Aids and lollipops. For little kids, it may help to distract them or hold their hand and let them squeeze when they get pricked.

Amy Lynn's comments:

Typically a dose of Tylenol following the shot will relieve any discomfort from the shot. If the area swells or bruises, an ice pack helps sometimes. But the biggest help for young children is a really fun, brightly colored band-aid! That typically stops any tears!

37. Should I give my child something to prevent fever or pain?

When your child is given shots in the clinic or doctor's office, you should ask your doctor whether you should give your child a non-aspirin pain reliever. Aspirin should not be used for relief of pain or fever in this situation because aspirin can rarely cause a severe disease in children if it is given to a child with certain types of viral infections. If any medication is used, the two most

Aspirin should not be used for relief of pain or fever in this situation because aspirin can rarely cause a severe disease in children if it is given to a child with certain types of viral infections.

Acetaminophen

A medicine often given to reduce pain and fever. Tylenol is a common brand name for this drug.

Ibuprofen

A medicine often given to reduce pain and fever. Advil and Motrin are common brand names for this drug.

frequently recommended are **acetaminophen** (Tylenol or other brands) or **ibuprofen** (brand names include Motrin, Advil, etc.). Always check with your doctor to make sure you know the correct dose of these medicines to give, depending on your child's weight and which preparation of the medicine you have, and to clarify how and when to use these medicines. A cool wet cloth can help lessen any redness, soreness, or swelling at the site of the shots. If your child has any concerning reaction, you should contact your doctor or seek medical attention.

Amy Lynn's comments:

I typically wait to see if they need it—most of the time we have not seen any fever or pain from the shots.

38. What do I do if my child misses some shots?

Vaccines are recommended to be given in a series of shots over a scheduled period of time. This schedule was created to try to optimize the development of immunity against certain diseases at certain ages. It is not uncommon for one or more shots to be missed due to delays in appointments or illness at the time of administration. In general, it is not a problem if a shot is missed, in that no additional shots (above the number recommended for the entire shot series) need to be given. However, it is strongly recommended that your child be brought up-to-date on the shots as soon as possible to help them be protected. There are specific schedules for "catch up" immunizations in certain circumstances where there has been a delay in immunizations. Your doctor can help your child get back on recommended schedule.

Amy Lynn's comments:

Talk with your pediatrician and they will figure out the best way to "make up" the shots.

39. How can I keep track of the vaccines my child has already received?

Currently, there is no central location or agency in the United States which keeps children's vaccination records. Every time your child gets a vaccine, the doctors and clinic staff are required to write down specific information about the vaccine. Federal agencies require that the doctor writes down the date the vaccine was given, the vaccine and the manufacturer, the lot number of the vaccine, the name and address of the clinic or office where the vaccine was given, the date the Vaccine Information Statement (VIS) was given to the parent or patient, and the date the VIS was published. In addition, the American Academy of Pediatrics suggests that doctors record the site and route of administration for the vaccine, the vaccine expiration date, and a written statement indicating the VIS was given and discussed. This is usually more information than the parent or patient needs, and often your child's doctor will give you an immunization card with the vaccine and date given listed for you to keep for your records. Your child's doctor's office or clinic should keep their copy of this immunization record, but it may not be kept permanently. Your child's school usually requires a vaccine record at the time of enrollment, but it is often kept for only a limited time after your child graduates from or leaves that school.

In most states, it is the responsibility of the parent to provide vaccine records to a school or health department. For children who have moved or changed health care providers, it is often a challenge to keep records accurate and current. As a parent, you should make sure your child's current doctor or clinic is sent or given a copy of all your child's past immunizations in order to maintain an accurate record for your child.

Some doctors have electronic records which keep this information up-to-date. An accurate record can be prepared for you when you need to supply a school, camp, or daycare with your child's immunization record. Often the doctor will give you a vaccine card to keep which lists each vaccine and the date your child received that vaccine. There are several styles of immunization records. One example, which can be printed for your own use, can be accessed at *http://www.immunize.org/catg.d/p2022.pdf*. A sample immunization record is shown in **Figure 1**. The website on the link just given also contains information about how the form is completed and how to interpret abbreviations used for these vaccines and their administration. Some computer software programs are designed to help parents create and maintain health records, including immunization records, for the entire family. One example of these programs, Health ePal, can be accessed free of charge from the Children's Hospital of Philadelphia website at *http://www.chop.edu/healthepal/download/index.shtml*.

In some states, computerized information systems which collect vaccine histories and help ensure timely administration of vaccines for children are being developed.

In some states, computerized information systems which collect vaccine histories and help ensure timely administration of vaccines for children are being developed. These systems are called **Vaccine Registries**. Such registries are helpful to parents as the system keeps a complete electronic record of each child's vaccine history and allows for easy notification from the doctor when appointments for immunization should be scheduled to keep immunizations current. The registries can also be used to see what percent of children in the practice or in the entire registry are up-to-date on any vaccine of interest. Larger registries are being developed, and there are ongoing discussions about the feasibility of creating a national registry for childhood vaccines.

Vaccine Registries

Computerized information systems which collect vaccine histories and help ensure timely administration of vaccines for children.

Amy Lynn's comments:

Most pediatricians have an immunization record booklet that you can take to each visit and they update it with each vaccine the child receives—it makes for a great place to keep all the information in a small booklet that you can use as proof of vaccines.

40. Vaccines are expensive! What if I can't pay for vaccines for my child?

Vaccines vary in cost, but the sum total price is expensive. If your child is covered under your or someone's health insurance, the cost of the vaccines is usually covered (after the deductible is met and possibly with a co-pay). However, there are multiple clinics which can provide the vaccines for free if you are eligible. In 1994, the **Vaccines for Children (VFC) Program** became operational. The VFC Program helps families of children who, due to financial reasons, may not otherwise have access to vaccines. The program provides free vaccines to the doctors who serve these children. Children through 18 years of age who are Medicaid-eligible, uninsured, an American Indian or Alaskan Native, or who are underinsured are eligible for the program. The **State Children's Health Insurance Program (SCHIP),** known as Title XXI, also enables states to expand health insurance coverage for uninsured children so that more children may be eligible for VFC. In this program, the vaccines are free, although you may need to pay a small fee for giving the vaccine. Most vaccines are available in this program. You can contact your doctor or your local health department to inquire about the closest VFC provider.

Amy Lynn's comments:

Check with your local health department—there are organizations that provide free or reduced-fee vaccines.

The VFC Program helps families of children who, due to financial reasons, may not otherwise have access to vaccines. The program provides free vaccines to the doctors who serve these children.

Vaccines for Children (VFC) Program

A federal program which helps families who have difficulty paying for vaccines to obtain vaccines for their children.

State Children's Health Insurance Program (SCHIP)

A program, also known as Title XXI, which helps states to expand health insurance coverage for uninsured children so that more children may be eligible for the Vaccines for Children program.

Vaccine Administration Record for Children and Teens

Patient Name _____ Date of Birth _____
Chart Number _____

Vaccine	Date Given	Site	Mfr. and Lot	Expiration Date	Consent	Provider	VIS Date
DTaP #1							
DTaP #2							
DTaP #3							
DTaP #4							
DTaP #5							
TdaP							
HIB #1							
HIB #2							
HIB #3							
HIB #4							
IPV #1							
IPV #2							
IPV #3							
IPV #4							
HEP B #1							
HEP B #2							
HEP B #3							
MMR #1							
MMR #2							
VAR #1							
VAR #2							
PCV7 #1							
PCV7 #2							
PCV7 #3							
PCV7 #4							
HEP A #1							
HEP A #2							
MEN							
HPV #1							
HPV #2							
HPV #3							
ROTA #1							
ROTA #2							
ROTA #3							
FLU							
FLU							
FLU							
FLU							
FLU							

Figure 1 Sample Immunization Record

PART FOUR

The Vaccine Schedule for Children

Which vaccines are recommended for children?

Are all of these vaccines required?
Does my child have to get these to attend school?

Does my child need a vaccine if he has already
had the disease it prevents?

More . . .

41. Which vaccines are recommended for children?

Vaccines are tested to determine the optimum dosage schedule to provide maximum efficacy and safety. There are recommended ages for giving each vaccine. There is some flexibility, in that if your child misses a dose she can catch up later, but the vaccines are not usually given earlier than scheduled. Your child's doctor can give you more information on any needed changes in the recommended schedule.

The 2008 routine childhood immunization schedule is shown in **Figure 2**. This schedule is updated at least yearly if not twice a year. Vaccine recommendations for children are issued primarily by two national groups, the U.S. Public Health Service's Advisory Committee on Immunization Practices (ACIP) and the American Academy of Pediatrics (AAP) Committee on Infectious Diseases. To access the most recent schedule and policy statements on vaccines, you can access the AAP website at *www.immunize.org/aap* or the ACIP website at *www.immunize.org/acip*.

42. Are all of these vaccines required? Does my child have to get these to attend school?

All states have mandated immunization requirements for children attending schools and daycares. However, in many states, **exemptions** are granted for medical, religious, or personal reasons. Medical exemptions are granted if your doctor believes your child should not receive a vaccine due to a weakened immune system, prior severe reaction to a vaccine, or other medical reason. All states accept medical exemptions. Religious exemptions are granted if the use of vaccines is against your religious beliefs. Only a couple of states do not accept this type of exemption. Personal reasons or personal

Exemptions

In reference to vaccines, the term exemption denotes an official exception to the requirement for giving a child a vaccine.

choice is accepted as an exemption in many, but not all, states. Regardless of the type of exemption, the parent or guardian must usually provide a signed written objection to the school or daycare, and sometimes this may need to be updated yearly. If there are questions about whether you can legally use a specific type of exemption, contact your school system, daycare, or local health department. Your child should not be excluded from school, although if there is an outbreak or concern of an outbreak of a vaccine-preventable disease, your child may be excluded from that school or facility for a period of time until there is no further public health threat.

The CDC vaccine website and other vaccine websites have information on vaccine requirements and exemptions listed by state. However, the most updated recommendations should be easily obtained by contacting your local school board.

43. Does my child need a vaccine if he has already had the disease it prevents?

If your child has already had the disease which the vaccine to be administered is designed to prevent, you need to discuss this with your doctor. For some diseases, if your child had a documented natural infection with that **pathogen**, a vaccine may not be necessary. However, for some diseases, especially diseases in which many different types of the microorganism can cause disease and not yield protection against all types, the vaccine may still be needed. If the disease was not confirmed to be due to a specific microorganism, your child's doctor may advise the use of the vaccine anyway. Sometimes obtaining a blood sample from your child to test for antibodies against a certain bacterium or virus will be sufficient to confirm prior protection.

For some diseases, if your child had a documented natural infection with that pathogen, a vaccine may not be necessary.

Pathogen

A microorganism which can cause infection or disease.

Vaccine	Birth	1 Month	2 Months	4 Months	6 Months	12 Months	15 Months	18 Months	19–23 Months	2–3 Years	4–6 Years	7–10 Years	11–12 Years	13–18 Years
Hepatitis B	X	X				X								
Rotavirus			X	X	X									
Diphtheria, Tetanus, Pertussis			X	X	X		X				X		X	
Haemophilus influenzae type B			X	X	X	X								
Pneumococcal			X	X	X	X								
Poliovirus			X	X	X						X			
Influenza						X (Yearly)								
Measles, Mumps, Rubella						X					X			
Varicella						X					X			
Hepatitis A							X							
Meningococcal													X	
Human Papillomavirus													X 3-Dose Series	

This schedule indicates the recommended ages for routine administration of the vaccines recommended for children in the United States as of January 1, 2008. For further details on the vaccines and schedule for administration, please refer to the text as well as to the official current vaccine schedule which can be accessed at the following CDC Website: http://www.cdc.gov/vaccines/recs/schedules/default.htm.

Figure 2 Recommended Immunization Schedule for Children (United States, 2008)

PART FIVE

Vaccines in the First 6 Months of Life

What is the DTaP (diphtheria, tetanus, acellular pertussis) vaccine?

I heard that the old pertussis vaccine could cause severe side effects. Is the current vaccine safer?

There are still outbreaks of whooping cough (pertussis). Does this mean the vaccine is ineffective?

More . . .

44. What is the DTaP (diphtheria, tetanus, acellular pertussis) vaccine?

The DTaP vaccine for infants and young children is a combination vaccine against three important diseases, diphtheria, tetanus (lockjaw), and pertussis (whooping cough).

Diphtheria is caused by bacteria called *Corynebacterium diphtheriae*. Although there were more than 150,000 cases and more than 15,000 deaths in the United States in the early 1900s, now we rarely see this severe disease due mainly to widespread use of the vaccine. People are the only source of this type of bacteria, which lives in the mouth, nose and throat of infected individuals. It is usually spread by cough or sneeze, but can be spread from contact with the rash which occurs in some types of diphtheria.

The first symptoms of diphtheria are often sore throat and fever. A membrane can eventually develop over the back of the throat. Eventually it can lead to severe swelling in the neck (called "bull neck") with blockage of the upper airway. Sometimes, diphtheria presents instead with a rash or infection of the eye or ear. The bacteria which cause diphtheria can make a toxin which can cause heart failure or paralysis. People with diphtheria are often quite ill, and one of every ten people with the disease die. Doctors can give an antitoxin and antibiotics to try to fight the infection and the effects of the toxin.

Tetanus is more common in warmer climates and during warmer months. It is not contagious.

Tetanus, or "lockjaw," is a disease which affects the nervous system and is caused by the bacterium *Clostridium tetani*. In the United States, we still see up to 50 cases per year, although this is significantly decreased from the early to mid 1900s. Tetanus is more common in warmer climates and during warmer months. It is not contagious. The bacteria live in dirt and manure, and usually enter the body through the skin, especially in deep cuts, wounds, or bites.

Tetanus usually presents 1–2 weeks after infection (but can start sooner) with the gradual onset of headache and irritability. Soon the classic muscle spasms of tetanus start to occur and become more severe. These spasms occur in jaw muscles, causing "lockjaw" or trismus, but also in muscles of the neck, arms, legs, and most muscle groups. The spasms are aggravated by any external stimulus, such as touch or a sudden noise. The cause of these effects on muscles and nerves is a toxin produced by the bacteria. Children with tetanus usually require hospitalization for a few weeks, often in the intensive care unit. Ten to twenty percent of tetanus patients die. Doctors can use antibiotics and an antibody preparation made to fight the toxin, but supportive care is just as important.

Pertussis, or whooping cough, is caused by bacteria called *Bordetella pertussis*. Pertussis is still quite common in the United States, with more than 25,000 cases reported in recent years. The highest rates are found in infants younger than 6 months and in children 10–14 years old; however, it is found in people of all ages. In the past, the frequency of pertussis used to increase then decrease every few years, but now it occurs at a relatively stable rate year to year. People are the only source of these bacteria. It is very contagious and is spread mainly by coughing and sneezing.

Symptoms of pertussis begin with runny nose and cold symptoms for 1–2 weeks. Since these symptoms do not usually make people think of pertussis, it usually goes undiagnosed at this point. This is unfortunate, because this is the time when the person is most contagious to others. After this stage of illness, the cough starts. The typical whooping cough consists of frequent episodes of rapid, repeated cough, followed by a large inhaled breath, which sounds like a whoop. Infants and young children are less likely to have the typical sound of a whoop, but are more likely to have problems breathing. Children this age can have episodes of gasping and periods where they stop breathing, called apnea. Sudden death has been reported. Children are also more likely to get pneumonia (20%), and 2% can have seizures. People recover slowly, and the cough can last for weeks to months. The diagnosis is confirmed with tests done from a swab from deep in the nose. Antibiotics are usually given, not as much to help the symptoms as to try to limit spread of the infection to others.

A combination vaccine for these three infectious diseases is recommended for all children. The vaccine is given at 2, 4, 6, 15–18 months, and then at 4–6 years of age. The vaccine used since the early 1990s is called **DTaP**, for diphtheria, tetanus, and acellular pertussis. The parts active against diphtheria and tetanus are really toxoids, or inactivated toxins. The acellular pertussis part of the vaccine has only part of the bacterium. It is a killed vaccine. One third of children may have a local reaction at the site of the immunization. It may be tender, red, and swollen. Fever, usually low-grade, can be seen, and children may seem fussy and not have the best appetite after getting the vaccine. The local reaction and fever are more common with the fourth and fifth vaccines. The vaccine works well; it is thought to be more than 80% effective for pertussis, 95% effective against diphtheria, and almost always effective against tetanus. However, a booster form of the vaccine is recommended at least every ten years and sometimes sooner if children have a serious wound which puts them at greater risk for tetanus.

DTaP

The diphtheria, tetanus, acellular pertussis vaccine recommended for children at 2, 4, 6, 15–18 months, and 4–6 years of age.

Children with minor illnesses such as a cold can safely receive the DTaP vaccine. If your child has a more severe illness, the vaccine should usually be delayed until recovery from the illness. Children who had either a life-threatening allergic reaction associated with the DTaP, or who experienced any disease associated with the brain or central nervous system within 6 days after receiving a previous dose of DTaP, should not receive this vaccine. If your child had a seizure, an episode of prolonged (>3 hours) crying, or temperature >105 after a previous dose of DTaP, you should discuss with your child's doctor whether the vaccine should be continued.

Other forms of the vaccine are given to certain children. A vaccine called **DT** is still made to give to children under 7 years old who should not take the pertussis part of the vaccine due to concern of prior reaction (see answer to next question). The **Td** vaccine is given to children older than 7 years of age for booster vaccines as needed. It has a smaller amount of the diphtheria to avoid adverse reactions, and normal amount of the tetanus. In 2005, a new vaccine was approved for teenagers called **Tdap**. It has the normal amount of tetanus with smaller amounts of both diphtheria and pertussis.

DT

A diphtheria-tetanus vaccine available for children under age 7 years who should not take the pertussis part of the vaccine due to concern arising from a prior reaction.

Td

The tetanus-diphtheria vaccine given to children older than age 7 years for booster vaccines as needed.

Tdap

A combination vaccine against tetanus, diphtheria, and acellular pertussis approved in 2005 for use in teenagers and some adults.

45. I heard that the old pertussis vaccine could cause severe side effects. Is the current vaccine safer?

Before 1996, the vaccine used for routine immunization was the DTP vaccine. The pertussis part of the vaccine was called a "whole-cell" vaccine because it contained killed whole bacteria. This vaccine was considered effective and generally safe, but a higher rate of adverse effects was reported with its use. The side effects were still not common, but included continuous crying for more than three hours and sometimes higher fever. Seizures occurred in some infants and were thought to be associated with the higher fever in most cases. There were several reports of infants having brain damage and it was unclear if the vaccine was the cause of that complication. The new acellular vaccine, DTaP, was developed and put into use in the 1990s. This vaccine has a much decreased frequency of adverse effects compared with the older DTP. The DTP is no longer in use in the United States.

46. There are still outbreaks of whooping cough (pertussis). Does this mean the vaccine is ineffective?

The pertussis vaccine is very effective in preventing severe disease due to pertussis but does not totally prevent infection. Many immunized people can become infected with pertussis and have either no symptoms or mild cold symptoms. This is often not even diagnosed as pertussis due to the mild symptoms. These individuals can, however, easily transmit the infection to others who are more susceptible, especially children in the same household. A larger number of cases of more severe disease in teenagers and adults have also been recently reported, which led to the recommendations for use of the new vaccine Tdap as a booster vaccine to help boost immunity to pertussis in teenagers and adults.

Mary Ellen's comments:

During my career, there has been resurgence in pertussis infections. Interesting to see how bacteria can reinvent themselves, causing infections in older patients.

47. Why are different diphtheria, tetanus, and pertussis vaccines used for older children?

Many years ago it was noted that children over 7 years of age, as well as adults, experienced a stronger adverse reaction to the diphtheria part of the vaccine if the same vaccine used for infants and young children was used for immunization. Therefore, the Td vaccine was developed for use as the booster vaccine. The amount of diphtheria toxoid in the Td Vaccine is less than one third the amount of diphtheria toxoid in the DTaP Vaccine. For children (or adults) who had the initial vaccine series as an infant, the smaller amount of diphtheria vaccine component worked just as well at boosting immunity but caused fewer reactions. Likewise, the new vaccine Tdap has lower amounts of the diphtheria toxoid as well as lower amounts of the pertussis vaccine, which produces fewer adverse reactions. Immunity against diphtheria, pertussis, and tetanus wanes, or decreases, as people age, and these booster vaccines are needed to boost your immunity against these three diseases. The vaccines described above create this boosted immunity with fewer side effects from the vaccine itself.

48. What is the polio vaccine?

Poliovirus is the name of the virus that causes polio, a disease which can be complicated by paralysis. In the early 1900s, the United States had an epidemic in which more than 27,000 people became paralyzed and 6,000 died. With the use of effective vaccines, the last case of actual polio in the United States was in 1979. Rarely, we still see cases of **VAPP—vaccine-associated paralytic polio**, a disease caused by the older live virus

Vaccine-associated paralytic polio (VAPP)

A type of polio which was associated with use of the older live virus vaccine which is no longer used in the United States.

71

vaccine no longer used in the United States. Usually infections were more common in the summer and fall. The virus is found only in people, usually in the throat and intestines. The virus could be found in the stool of someone who had the infection for several weeks to a few months. It could be passed on to others by contact with infected fluids from respiratory secretions or stool. There are three types of poliovirus, all of which are in the vaccine.

Poliovirus infections were more common in children. Most infections (95%) did not cause any symptoms. Sometimes children had a mild sore throat, fever and cold symptoms, with occasional stiff neck or back and leg pain. The infection caused severe leg pains followed by paralysis in only a very small percentage of children. The paralysis was usually in the legs, but could affect other muscles, including muscles needed for breathing. Long ago, when polio was a common illness, machines called **Iron Lungs** were used to try to save people with severe illness affecting their ability to breathe. Today there is still no specific drug treatment which is effective against the virus.

Currently only one poliovirus vaccine is used in the United States, the **IPV**, or **inactivated polio vaccine**. This vaccine has killed virus from each of the three types of poliovirus. It is given in four doses, at 2, 4, 6–18 months, and last at 4–6 years of age. This vaccine is very safe, with the main side effect being occasional soreness and redness where the vaccine was given. It is very effective, with studies showing it works in preventing infection 99% of the time.

If your child has a minor illness such as a cold, the polio vaccine can still be given. However, children with more

Iron Lungs

Machines used in the past to treat people with severe polio who were unable to breathe without assistance.

Inactivated polio vaccine (IPV)

The current polio vaccine used in the United States. The vaccine has killed virus from each of the three types of poliovirus.

severe illnesses should usually delay immunization with the polio vaccine until after they have recovered from the illness. Any child who has had a severe allergic reaction with a prior polio vaccine should not receive the vaccine. Also, children who have had a severe allergic reaction to any of the antibiotics neomycin, streptomycin, or polymyxin should not receive the polio vaccine.

Mary Ellen's comments:

Polio was feared when I was a child. Consequently, I was kept indoors during the summer to avoid getting polio. The polio vaccine certainly gave the freedom of summer back!

49. I remember the old polio vaccine you took by mouth. Why don't we use that vaccine now?

A live virus vaccine for poliovirus was used in the United States for many years. It was a liquid which could be swallowed, squirted in the mouth, or even put on a sugar cube to take. The vaccine had all three types of the poliovirus which were live, not killed, but changed to a weakened form of the virus. The vaccine was very effective in preventing the actual virus infection, but sometimes the weakened virus in the vaccine caused a disease called VAPP, vaccine-associated paralytic polio. From the late 1980s to mid-1990s, about 8 cases of VAPP occurred in the United States. In order to prevent this form of polio, the decision was made to switch to using only the current killed vaccine. Since the year 2000, only the killed IPV has been given as a vaccine in the United States. Cases of VAPP have seemed to disappear, although not totally. Because the **OPV** is still used in many other countries, people traveling to other countries can sometimes come in contact with

Oral Polio Vaccine (OPV)

A live polio vaccine no longer used in the United States but still in use in other countries.

the OPV virus. In 2005, a person in the United States was diagnosed with VAPP with which he was infected when traveling to another country. Also, the same year, several children were found to have the vaccine virus strain but they had no symptoms. Therefore, until polio is eradicated in the world, it is important to continue immunization against polio.

50. What is the Hib (Haemophilus influenzae *Type B) vaccine*?

Haemophilus influenzae **type b** (Hib for short) is a bacterium which causes a wide variety of infections, some of which can be very serious. Prior to use of the vaccine, it was the most common cause of **meningitis** (infection of the lining or membranes around the brain) in young children. Hib infections were also a common cause of pneumonia, fever with bacteria in the bloodstream, and other serious diseases. Currently, we see the infections only in underimmunized children or in children too young for the vaccine. The bacteria live in the nose and sinuses and can be spread to others by coughing or sneezing. It often causes no symptoms in children if the bacteria stay in the nose and sinuses, but it can get into the bloodstream and cause illness. Other types of *Haemophilus influenzae* besides type b are still common causes of ear and sinus infections. The diseases caused by these other types are usually milder but, rarely, they can cause serious disease.

The range of diseases caused by Hib includes pneumonia, **bacteremia** (bacteria in the blood) with fever, meningitis, **epiglottitis** (a type of severe throat infection), skin

---

Haemophilus influenzae type b (Hib)

A bacterium which can cause a wide variety of infections in children, including pneumonia, bacteremia, meningitis, epiglottitis, and infection of the skin, joints, bones, and ears.

Meningitis

Infection of the lining or membranes around the brain.

Bacteremia

The presence of bacteria in the bloodstream.

Epiglottitis

Inflammation of the epiglottis, which is the structure at the base of the tongue which stops food from entering the trachea (windpipe).

infection, joint and bone infection, and ear infections. There are also other types of infections which are less common. Infections can be treated with antibiotics, but many of these infections are severe and can cause long term problems, and even death. Meningitis is one of the most severe, and many children have brain damage as a result of the infection.

Several brands of the Hib vaccine are used. All are killed vaccines made from parts of the bacteria. The first Hib conjugate vaccine was approved for use in 1988. Since that time, the number of serious infections due to Hib has decreased by 99%. The vaccine is very effective, and works 95–100% of the time in preventing serious Hib infections. Three or four shots are required, depending on the brand of vaccine used. It is given at 2, 4, 6, and then at 12–15 months of age. One brand of the Hib vaccine is somewhat different from the others. When the manufacturer of the PedvaxHIB vaccine tested their vaccine, they found that the vaccine had a good immune response without the 6-month dose. The resultant immunity to the different brands after completion of the vaccine series is all very similar, but the other brands include the 6-month shot. All Hib vaccines are considered safe, often with no side effects seen. When noted, the only reactions are usually mild tenderness and redness at the site of the shot.

Children with minor illnesses such as a cold can safely receive the Hib vaccine. If your child has a more severe illness, the vaccine should usually be delayed until recovery from the illness. The vaccine should also not be given to any infant less than 6 weeks of age or to any child who has experienced a life-threatening allergic reaction with a prior Hib vaccine.

Mary Ellen's comments:

The Hib vaccine caused the virtual disappearance of meningitis caused by that bacterium. Business in the microbiology lab dropped accordingly.

51. What is the pneumococcal vaccine?

Streptococcus pneumoniae

A common bacterium which causes many types of infections in children.

The bacterium **Streptococcus pneumoniae**, often called pneumococcus, is a very common cause of a variety of infections in children. (*Streptococcus pyogenes*, or Group A Strep, is the bacterium that causes "strep throat" and scarlet fever; it is related to but different from pneumococcus). Prior to the year 2000, when the current pneumococcal vaccine was introduced for use in infants, pneumococcus was the most common bacterial cause of severe invasive infections in children and the most common cause of ear infections. It is well known to cause meningitis, pneumonia, infections in the blood, sinusitis, **conjunctivitis** (eye infections) and a variety of

Conjunctivitis

An infection of the conjunctiva, the inner surface of the eyelid and outer surface of the eye.

other types of serious infections. Rates of infection are higher in infants, young children, and the elderly, and are also higher in certain ethnic groups and in anyone with certain chronic diseases (e.g., sickle cell anemia) or conditions which weaken the immune system. Although infections occur year round, they are mostly seen in winter months and in early spring. The bacteria live in the nasal passages and upper airways of many people and are usually spread by the respiratory route (coughing, sneezing). Antibiotics are used for treatment of infections, although some types of the bacterium are growing resistant to the usual antibiotics.

Prevnar

The killed pneumococcal vaccine used in infants and young children.

There are > 90 different types of pneumococcus, and the vaccine **Prevnar** has the 7 types which cause most invasive disease (80%) in young children. This is a killed vaccine. It is recommended to be given at 2, 4, 6, and 12–15 months of age. Local reactions with redness and soreness occur in 10–20% of children, often after the last dose. Some children have mild fever after the shot. The vaccine works very well. Since the vaccine's first use in 2000, serious invasive disease by all pneumococcus types has decreased by 80% and infections due to the 7 types in the vaccine have decreased by 90%.

As with most other vaccines, children with minor illnesses such as a cold can safely receive either of the pneumococcal vaccines. If your child has a more severe illness, the vaccine should usually be delayed until recovery from the illness. Children who have had a severe allergic reaction to a previous dose of the vaccine, or who are known to be allergic to any of the vaccine components should not receive the vaccine.

Mary Ellen's comments:

Serious S. pneumo *infections (e.g., sepsis, meningitis, mastoiditis) decreased significantly once the vaccine became available. There was still job security as a microbiology tech since ear and sinus infections seemed to march right along.*

52. Why are there two types of the pneumococcal vaccine?

Since 1977, a different vaccine for pneumococcus has been in use for immunizing selected children and adults at high risk of pneumococcal infections. This vaccine, called **Pneumovax**, is a type of vaccine called a polysaccharide vaccine. This type of vaccine is made by using the outer coat of the bacterium, the capsule, as part of the vaccine. Unfortunately, this type of vaccine does not work well in young children, but works very

Pneumovax

The pneumococcal vaccine for use in older children and adults.

well in older children and adults. Pneumovax contains parts of 23 different types of pneumococcus. This vaccine is still used as the pneumococcal vaccine given for immunizations in older children and adults.

53. Does my child need to get both types of the pneumococcal vaccine when he is older?

Pneumococcal vaccines are not routinely given to healthy children above age 2 years or to healthy young adults, because the risk of significant pneumococcal disease is not as high in these age groups. The vaccine may be given to elderly individuals who are more susceptible to having severe disease due to the pneumococcus. Children and adults with certain chronic diseases (e.g. sickle cell disease), or conditions which cause a weakened immune system, are considered at higher risk and should get booster doses of a pneumococcal vaccine. Usually the vaccine given to older children and adults is Pneumovax; however, studies are underway to see if there is any benefit from giving the vaccine Prevnar followed by Pneumovax as a booster to some people to get better immunity.

54. Is the pneumococcal vaccine the same as the pneumonia vaccine?

Often people call the pneumococcal vaccine the pneumonia vaccine. Since the pneumococcus is a major cause of bacterial pneumonia, and use of the vaccine can decrease the risk of pneumonia due to these bacteria, this title conveys some truth. However, it must be remembered that many different bacteria, viruses, and other infectious agents can cause pneumonia. In addition to the pneumo-coccus, bacteria such as *Staphylococcus aureus*, *Streptococcus pyogenes* ("Group A Strep"), Mycoplasma (one cause of "walking pneumonia"), *Mycobacterium tuberculosis* ("TB"), as well as influenza and other common childhood viruses can all cause pneumonia. The pneumococcal vaccine is not capable of preventing pneumonia due to any of these other germs. Some of these other causes of pneumonia, for instance influenza, can be prevented by use of other vaccines. Therefore, the pneumococcal vaccine can be considered to be a "pneumonia vaccine," but it certainly cannot prevent all types of pneumonia and it can prevent other types of diseases.

55. What is the Hepatitis B vaccine?

Hepatitis B Virus (HBV) is one of several viruses that can cause hepatitis, an infection and/or inflammation of the liver. More than 1 million people in the United States are chronically infected with HBV. Every year 4–5,000 people in the United States die from hepatitis B. It can be acquired at any age, and a mother who is infected with hepatitis B can infect her baby at birth. The virus is in the blood and body fluids of an infected person and is usually transmitted to others at birth from an infected mother or by unprotected sex, sharing nee-dles, or getting a needle stick. Now, donated blood is tested for the virus, but historically it was sometimes acquired from blood transfusions.

Some people who get hepatitis B are totally asymptomatic and do not realize they are ill. Others have only nausea and fatigue, and others have **jaundice** (yellow skin and eyes), dark urine, vomiting and diarrhea, and abdominal pains. Hepatitis B Virus is a type of hepatitis virus which

Hepatitis B Virus (HBV)

One of several viruses that can cause infec-tion and/or inflam-mation of the liver.

Jaundice

A yellow color of the skin and eyes, usu-ally seen in people who have hepatitis, an inflammation or infection of the liver.

can cause chronic infections. Some people infected with the virus recover without complications, while others go on to have chronic infection. Chronic infection occurs in >90% of infants who get it from their mother, in 25–50% of children ages 1 to 5 years, and in 2–6% of older children and adults. People with chronic infection can have **cirrhosis** (scarring) of their liver, liver cancer, or liver failure as a result of the chronic infection.

Cirrhosis

Extensive scarring of the liver usually seen with chronic hepatitis.

The Hepatitis B Vaccine is a killed vaccine made from a small part of the virus. The usual schedule is a series of three shots in the muscle, usually at birth, then 1–4 months, then 6–18 months. There is some flexibility with the schedule and older children may complete the series sooner than 6 months. The vaccine has few side effects with the most common being soreness in the muscle where it was given. The vaccine in children has a 98–100% efficacy rate.

Children with minor illnesses such as a cold can safely receive the Hepatitis B Vaccine. If your child has a more severe illness, the vaccine should usually be delayed until recovery from the illness. Children who have had a severe allergic reaction to a previous dose of the vaccine or who are known to be allergic to any of the vaccine components, including yeast, should not receive the vaccine. Pregnancy is not a contraindication to receiving the Hepatitis B Vaccine.

56. Why do some babies get the first dose at birth and some later?

For some time the initial dose of the vaccine for infants was given either at birth or at one of the first visits to the pediatrician. If the infant's mother had documented infection with hepatitis B, it was always recommended that the vaccine be given, along with specific antibody (called **hepatitis B immune globulin**), right after birth. Recommendations changed several years ago to encourage the use of the vaccine right after birth before the infant left the hospital in order to ensure maximum protection of the infant. Currently, the only exception to this is for a premature infant whose mother does not have hepatitis B; in this case, people recommend waiting until age two months for this infant to receive the first dose of vaccine. If a premature infant's mother does have hepatitis B, the infant should still get the vaccine soon after birth.

Hepatitis B immune globulin

Specific antibody against Hepatitis B Virus. Often called "H-BIG," it is given with vaccine in certain circumstances to prevent transmission of this virus infection.

57. What is the rotavirus vaccine?

Rotavirus is a common, highly contagious virus that is an important cause of severe diarrhea in children. Almost all children in the United States have had this virus infection by age five, and infections are very common in infants. Prior to the vaccine, approximately 70,000 children were hospitalized every year due to rotavirus illness. The virus causes large outbreaks of disease in the winter and spring, but can be seen any season of the year. Rotavirus is in the stool of infected children and is easily spread to other people on contaminated hands and surfaces. There are different types of the virus, and children can get repeated episodes of illness.

It is difficult to predict how rotavirus will affect your child. The infection may cause no symptoms, mild illness, or severe symptoms due to significant diarrhea and vomiting. The illness usually begins with fever, stomach upset, and vomiting, but soon progresses to watery diarrhea. Young children can have as many as 20 watery stools daily with severe rotavirus illnesses. The illness can last from three to nine days. More severe disease is due to loss of enough body fluids to cause dehydration. Signs of dehydration include dry mouth, sunken eyes, decrease in the amount of urine, and eventually extreme sleepiness or lethargy. There is no cure for rotavirus, but the most important part of supportive care is to give enough fluids to prevent and treat dehydration.

In February of 2006, the FDA approved the rotavirus vaccine called **RotaTeq**, and in April of 2008 the FDA approved a second rotavirus vaccine called **Rotarix**. These vaccines consist of live viruses which have been weakened so that they do not cause significant illness. The RotaTeq vaccine is given to infants by mouth at approximately age 2 months, 4 months, and 6 months. Rotarix was approved for use in a two-dose series, at two and four months of age. Both vaccines are usually well-tolerated, and the only common side effects reported are mild diarrhea and vomiting. Studies have shown that RotaTeq prevents about 70% of all rotavirus infections and prevents almost 100% of episodes of severe diarrhea caused by rotavirus. Studies indicate that the efficacy of the newer Rotarix vaccine is similar.

Infants with minor illnesses such as a cold can safely receive the rotavirus vaccines. However, if your baby has a more severe illness, or has an illness with vomiting and/or diarrhea, the vaccine should usually be delayed until recovery from the illness. Infants who have had severe allergic reaction to a previous dose of the rotavirus vaccine or who are known to be allergic to any of the vaccine components should not receive the vaccine. Infants with a weakened immune system due to HIV infection, steroids, or drugs used to treat certain types of cancers should also not receive the vaccine. If any infant

RotaTeq

A rotavirus vaccine approved in 2006 for use in young infants.

Rotarix

A rotavirus vaccine approved in 2008 for use in young infants.

has been previously diagnosed with an intestinal problem called intussusception (see question 58), that infant should not receive this vaccine. Finally, for infants who have either recently received a blood product or who have other types of intestinal illness, your child's doctor can help decide whether the rotavirus vaccine should be given.

58. Did this vaccine cause complications in some babies? I thought it was not used anymore.

The first vaccine approved for the prevention of rotavirus disease, **RotaShield**, was approved for use in the United States in the late 1990s. However, in a short time this vaccine was removed from the market due to concerns it might increase the risk of a bowel disorder seen in infants called **intussusception**. This vaccine is no longer on the market and is not available for use.

Intussusception is a blockage or twisting of the intestine which can be life-threatening. Although it can happen at any age, it most commonly occurs in the first year of life. It is reported in about 1 of every 2,000 infants. Cases of intussusception can occur with some types of viral infection or with an enlarged part of the intestine (e.g. a large lymph node in the bowel), but in most cases no cause is discovered. Infants with this disease become ill and have vomiting, stomach pain, periods of intermittent crying (associated with the pain), and sometimes blood in the stool. Treatment for intussusception can involve giving a special enema with air or fluid under pressure, but may require surgery if the bowel does not correct with the enema. If treatment is prompt, the infants usually do well and recover without complications.

RotaShield

The first rotavirus vaccine approved for use in the United States.

Intussusception

A blockage or twisting of the intestine which can be life-threatening.

Further review of the reports of infants who developed intussusception with the RotaShield vaccine has led to uncertainty as to whether this vaccine caused a greater number of cases of the disorder than could be expected to occur naturally. However, due to the possibility of this occurring, the drug companies producing the two current rotavirus vaccines have done very large studies to try to detect any increase in the number of cases of intussusception with the use of their rotavirus vaccines. For instance, RotaTeq was tested in a study of 70,000 children, and there was no evidence that the vaccine caused this disorder. In addition, both the companies and the CDC are continuing larger scale studies to follow infants immunized with the vaccines to make sure there is no increased risk of this disorder. Additional rotavirus vaccines are also in various stages of development, and drug companies studying and producing these vaccines will be expected to prove that their vaccine has no increased risk of intussusception before the vaccine is approved for use.

59. My baby was late starting this vaccine and my doctor said not to start it. Why?

The series of two or three doses (dependent upon which vaccine is given) of rotavirus vaccine is started in young infants at about age 2 months. This vaccine schedule is thought to be the best in order to prevent severe rotavirus diarrhea in young infants. Although infants and children of any age can have some symptoms with the virus infection, the worst disease and the most complications are seen in young infants who get this infection. The vaccine has not been well studied in infants who were delayed in starting the vaccine. Since no one can be certain whether the vaccine might cause more adverse effects, such as intussusception or other bowel disease, or be less effective when started in older infants and children, the approval for use was for starting the vaccine by a certain age in early infancy. Therefore, if your baby does not get the first dose of the vaccine by a certain age, your child's doctor might not start the vaccine series at all. It is possible that further studies will be done to confirm that the vaccine is as safe and effective when started later, and that the age range for starting the vaccine will be changed.

60. Will the rotavirus vaccine stop my baby from getting diarrhea?

The rotavirus vaccines have proven to be very effective for preventing severe rotavirus disease and in reducing the amount of diarrhea and the number of hospitalizations due to rotavirus. Studies have shown that the vaccine prevents about 70% of all rotavirus infections and prevents almost all episodes of severe diarrhea caused by rotavirus. However, immunized infants can still have mild diarrhea due to rotavirus. In addition, even the vaccine itself can cause mild diarrhea in some infants.

Diarrhea is a very common illness in infants and young children. Many different types of infections can result in diarrhea. Other types of viruses, including viruses which cause mostly cold symptoms, can cause diarrhea in some children. Infection with certain types of bacteria and other types of germs can also result in vomiting and diarrhea. Stools in infants may change consistency with changes in formula and with the introduction of new foods. Medications, especially antibiotics, commonly cause diarrhea. Rotavirus infection is a major cause of vomiting and diarrhea in infants and the use of effective vaccines is expected to have a significant impact on the health of infants. But probably your baby will have at least several episodes of diarrheal disease due to other causes during the first few years of life, and the rotavirus vaccine cannot prevent this.

PART SIX

Vaccines from Age 6 Months to 2 Years

At this age does my child need more doses
of some vaccines she has already received?

What is the influenza vaccine?

Why are there different types of influenza vaccines?

More . . .

61. At this age does my child need more doses of some vaccines she has already received?

Between the ages of 6 months and 2 years, some of the vaccines started earlier in infancy should be continued to get full protection from these vaccines. Vaccines for diphtheria, tetanus, pertussis, polio, *Haemophilus influenzae*, pneumococcus, hepatitis B, and rotavirus may need to be completed or continued during this time period. As these have been discussed in the previous section, please refer to the section on that specific vaccine or refer to the entire vaccine schedule shown in Figure 2.

62. What is the influenza vaccine?

True influenza is caused by one of the viruses called influenza virus. There are three different types of influenza virus, called influenza A, B, and C. Influenza A and B cause significant disease in people. Much confusion is caused by the fact that many other winter virus infections cause the same signs and symptoms as influenza, and often the illness is incorrectly attributed to that virus. Influenza causes more deaths in the United States than any other vaccine-preventable disease, about 36,000 deaths per year. Many of these deaths occur among the elderly, but children can also die from the disease. Influenza occurs in the winter months. It is very contagious, and is spread by coughing or sneezing or by direct contact with secretions from an infected person.

Influenza causes more deaths in the United States than any other vaccine-preventable disease, about 36,000 deaths per year.

The signs and symptoms of influenza often begin with mild cold-like symptoms, sore throat, headache, fever, and muscle aches. Vomiting and diarrhea can occur, but are actually unusual with true influenza and occur more often in younger children. Often the cough worsens and can turn into pneumonia. Infants may have a variety of symptoms ranging from those described above to a barking cough (an illness called **croup**), pneumonia, and severe illness with low blood pressure. Complications include pneumonia, which may be due to a second infection with bacteria, ear and sinus infections, inflammation of the heart, and even seizures or a severe infection of the brain called **encephalitis**. Several medicines exist which can be used to either treat or prevent influenza. Two drugs commonly used are **Tamiflu (oseltamivir)** and **Relenza (zanamavir)**. Tamiflu is available in liquid medicine or pills, while Relenza is given as an inhaled powder. To be effective for treatment, either drug must be used early in the illness and strains of influenza are getting resistant to these and other drugs.

There are different types of influenza vaccine, a killed vaccine given as a shot and a newer type of live virus vaccine (approved in 2003) which is sprayed into the nose. Each vaccine has a mixture of Influenza A and B viruses which may change in the vaccine every year. After age 6 months, the influenza vaccine is recommended yearly for children. The first time a child under the age of 9 years gets the vaccine two doses must be given one month apart. In 15–20% of children, the shot can cause a local reaction with some pain. Occasionally, a mild fever may occur. This vaccine is killed and is incapable of giving someone the influenza virus. The live weakened virus vaccine can give some children a fever and headache, and occasionally some abdominal pain or vomiting. It is unclear whether these symptoms are due to the virus itself. The effectiveness of the influenza vaccine depends on many factors, but especially if the type of viruses causing infections in a given year are the same types of virus in the vaccine. Both influenza

Croup

A respiratory illness, usually caused by a virus infection, which affects infants and young children.

Encephalitis

An infection of the brain. Patients with encephalitis may have headache, fever, sensitivity of the eyes to light and even seizures.

Tamiflu (Oseltamivir)

A medicine used for both treatment and prevention of influenza.

Relenza (Zanamavir)

A medicine used for both treatment and prevention of influenza.

vaccines can be effective, with the shot capable of being up to 70–90% effective in preventing influenza in healthy children and the live virus vaccine being >85% effective in young school aged children tested. However, during the influenza season in 2007 to 2008, the influenza viruses in the vaccine did not match the virus causing disease in most communities in the United States, and the vaccine was estimated to be only 44% effective.

In February of 2008, the Advisory Committee on Immunization Practices (ACIP) recommended that all children from age 6 months to 18 years of age receive an annual influenza vaccine. This group based its recommendation on several factors, including the good safety record and usual efficacy of the vaccine in this age group, the number of adverse effects and complications of influenza seen in this age group, and the expectation that immunization will reduce disease not only in the children, but also among household contacts and in the community. This new recommendation, unless changed, is to take effect no later than the 2009–2010 influenza season. This change in recommendation is expected to create challenges in the short term to ensure companies can supply enough vaccine and that there is an effective way to administer the vaccine to all children. At the time of publication of this book, discussions regarding implementation of this recommendation are ongoing.

The same general rules for vaccine administration used in other vaccines apply to the influenza vaccines. Children with minor illnesses such as a cold can safely receive either of the influenza vaccines; if your child has a more severe illness, though, the vaccine should usually be delayed until recovery from the illness. Children who have had a severe allergic reaction to a previous dose of the vaccine or who are known to be allergic to any of the vaccine components should not receive the vaccine. If your child has an allergy to eggs, these vaccines should be avoided. If your child has ever had a neurologic disease called **Guillain-Barre Syndrome**, only the killed vaccine should be considered and only after discussion with your child's doctor. The live virus influenza vaccine has more contraindications for use, including children with a weakened immune system, children on chronic aspirin therapy, and children with a variety of chronic or acute medical conditions affecting the lungs, heart, and other organ systems. Your child's doctor can discuss with you if your child is a candidate for the live virus vaccine.

63. Why are there different types of influenza vaccines?

The short answer to this question is that there are different types of influenza viruses, these viruses keep changing, and the best type of vaccine to give to people is unclear and depends on several factors.

There are several challenges to creating an effective vaccine against influenza. As mentioned previously, there are two main types of influenza virus, influenza A and B, which cause significant disease in people. Influenza A virus has different subtypes based on changes in two different proteins on the virus. The major challenge arises from the fact that these proteins keep changing, with both minor changes and major changes, the latter due to the viruses combining with another different influenza virus and "swapping" some of the proteins. You can be immune to one influenza virus, but as soon as its proteins change, you may no longer be immune.

Guillain-Barre Syndrome

A disease of the nervous system which usually presents with weakness of the legs and spreads to the arms and face.

If your child has an allergy to eggs, these influenza vaccines should be avoided. If your child has ever had a neurologic disease called Guillain-Barre Syndrome, only the killed vaccine should be considered and only after discussion with your child's doctor.

Scientists must make an educated guess every year as to which type of virus will exist in the community; this has to be done almost a year before the next influenza season to allow companies to make enough of the new virus vaccine. Sometimes the guess is correct and the vaccine works well to prevent influenza. But sometimes the guess is off and the vaccine is not very effective. In the 2007- 2008 flu season, the vaccine was, unfortunately, a poor match to the actual types of virus causing disease in the United States, and the effectiveness of the vaccine was low. Usually the vaccine is much more effective.

The live influenza virus vaccines recently developed were hoped to be even more effective than the killed vaccines. The live virus vaccines are sprayed into the nose and act more like the actual virus infection. In theory, this may cause better immunity to develop in the nose and respiratory tract, which may be more effective at preventing infection from the real influenza virus. However, not all children can take this type of live vaccine, and scientists are still trying to make improvements to create a more effective vaccine that all children can use.

64. I had the flu vaccine and then got the flu. Does this vaccine work?

A common story is that someone gets their influenza vaccine and then within a week or two has the signs and symptoms of influenza. The natural thoughts would be that the vaccine actually gave that person influenza disease. Usually the explanation is that the illness is due to a different winter virus which mimics the signs and symptoms of influenza but is not really influenza. Since influenza vaccines are given either at the beginning of or in the midst of the season of the year that we have the greatest number of other viral respiratory pathogens, many viruses infecting people in the community cause the same signs and symptoms as influenza.

However, sometimes the illness people get after receiving the influenza vaccine truly is influenza. Sometimes this occurs simply because the vaccine was given too late to build an immunity to that specific influenza virus. Another reason, as discussed previously, is that the vaccine was not very effective that year in giving protection against the type of influenza virus in the community. Immunization may provide some degree of immunity to modify the disease, or make the illness less severe, but not enough to prevent infection. In summary, although this phenomenon does certainly happen, most health care providers believe that the protection usually afforded by the vaccine is definitely worthwhile, and recommend following the current guidelines for vaccine administration.

Amy Lynn's comments:

From what I understand, the flu vaccine is a combination of the strands they predict will be present that year. Sometimes the selection is correct, sometimes it is off a little bit. However, with our experience, for the people who got the shot, if they did get the flu that year, it has been a much lighter case than anyone who did not get it.

65. What is the bird flu (avian influenza), and is there a vaccine for this?

Sometimes human influenza viruses can combine with animal influenza viruses, creating a new virus which has some components of both. In addition, some animal influenza viruses may acquire the ability to infect people. The "bird flu," or **avian influenza**, is a strain

Avian influenza

A strain of influenza virus that has caused a large number of infections and death in birds in Southeast Asia and now other parts of the world. It is able to spread to humans.

of the virus that has been infecting and killing a significant number of birds and poultry in Southeast Asia for the past ten years and has now spread to other areas of the world. Since 1997, it has been known that the virus is able to spread to people. As of mid-2008, there have been almost 400 cases of bird flu with 241 deaths confirmed in humans. Most human cases have been in Indonesia and other countries in Southeast Asia, but human cases have been documented in Africa and infected poultry have been detected in countries in Asia, Africa, and Europe.

The spread of this specific virus has been especially concerning because most people who acquired the bird flu have had severe disease. The clinical symptoms of bird flu may start like any type of influenza, but many people progress to severe breathing problems, pneumonia, and other severe complications. Worldwide, almost two thirds of people with confirmed bird flu have died from the infection. It is not clear whether some people may have milder illness and are not diagnosed with bird flu. Regardless, scientists are concerned that a pandemic, or worldwide epidemic, may occur with either this strain of bird flu or with a related or new strain of influenza to which no one is immune. Scientists are closely watching for the emergence of new strains of influenza and are constantly monitoring the types of this virus which are infecting both people and birds in various parts of the world. The current United States influenza vaccine is not designed to be protective against the bird flu, but scientists are trying to create an effective vaccine against this strain in case more widespread infection begins.

66. Why do you have to get the flu vaccine every year?

One of the challenges with the influenza vaccine described in the answer to question 64 is the constant change in the strains or types of influenza that appear in the United States every year. Sometimes the same type of influenza is back the next year, but often there are at least minor changes, and sometimes major changes, in the strain. The immunity provided by the vaccine against the previous strains may give little or no protection against the new types of virus. In addition, the immunity gained from the influenza vaccines is, unfortunately, not of long duration. Therefore, to provide the best protection, it is necessary to get the vaccine every year to boost your immunity to strains from prior vaccines as well as try to gain immunity to new strains.

To provide the best protection, it is necessary to get the flu vaccine every year to boost your immunity to strains from prior vaccines as well as try to gain immunity to new strains.

67. What is the MMR (measles, mumps, rubella) vaccine?

The MMR vaccine is a combination vaccine against three important diseases: measles, mumps, and rubella.

Measles is caused by the measles virus (also called rubeola virus). Before vaccine use in the United States, it caused an average of 450 deaths per year, and today still causes half a million deaths in the world each year. Currently, most of the average of 50 cases per year in the United States are due to travel and exposure of unvaccinated individuals. Historically, preschool and young school-age children were at the highest risk of getting the disease. It occurs mostly in late winter to spring. Spread occurs via respiratory secretions in the air—coughing and sneezing, or contact with infected secretions.

Eight to 12 days after infection, the signs and symptoms of measles start with runny nose, conjunctivitis (red eyes), cough and fever. A few days later, at the peak of the respiratory symptoms, the typical rash of measles erupts. It usually starts near the forehead around the scalp with flat or slightly raised red spots. The rash spreads to involve the face, upper trunk and arms, then lower trunk and legs. The rash becomes more confluent with time. Some children may get an ear infection, symptoms of croup (barking cough), and diarrhea with the disease. More severe illnesses, such as pneumonia, occur in 1 in 20 and encephalitis (brain infection) in 1 in 1,000 people with measles. There is no specific therapy for measles, but vitamin A is sometimes given to measles patients.

Mumps is caused by a virus of the same name as the disease—the mumps virus. Before the vaccine, there were more than 150,000 cases a year in the United States; but after vaccine use, the numbers have dropped to about 300 cases per year. However, following an initial case on a college campus in Iowa in late 2005, a multi-state outbreak with >5,000 cases occurred. Mumps often appears in winter and early spring but can occur any time of year. Infection rates are similar in males and females, but males are more likely to have complications. The respiratory secretions of a person with mumps are infectious three days before and up to nine days after symptoms begin. The virus is quite contagious, and 80—90% of unimmunized people living in the same house as a person with mumps will get mumps. As with measles, mumps is acquired after contact with infectious respiratory secretions.

Almost one third of people with mumps have only mild cold symptoms or no symptoms.

Almost one third of people with mumps have only mild cold symptoms or no symptoms. Two to three weeks after infection, children can have fever, headache, muscle aches, ear pain, fatigue, and decreased appetite. Often, within a day the classic swelling of salivary glands begins. The gland most often affected is the **parotid gland**, which is located at the jaw line just below the ear. The swelling is due to inflammation of one or more salivary glands. Complications can certainly occur. Fewer than 10% of children get meningitis or encephalitis with the virus infection. Permanent hearing loss can occur. Other complications include inflammation of the testes, ovaries or breasts.

Rubella, also called German measles or three-day measles, is caused by the rubella virus. Before use of the vaccine in the United States, there were epidemics every 6 to 9 years. In a major epidemic in the 1960s, 12.5 million people got the disease and 20,000 babies were born with congenital rubella syndrome, a severe complication in the baby of an infected pregnant mother. Since development of the vaccine, rubella levels have continued to drop and there is hope that the virus infection is gone from the United States. The virus is most prevalent in winter and spring, and is spread the same way as measles and mumps, by respiratory secretions.

In 25–50% of rubella infections there are no signs or symptoms of illness. The disease is usually mild, with fever and a mild rash on the face and trunk. Older children are more likely to get more swollen glands in the back of the neck as well as painful joints or arthritis. The biggest concern with rubella has always been when a pregnant woman gets infected during pregnancy. The virus can infect the fetus, and the baby can be born deaf or blind with heart and brain problems.

In the 1960s, separate vaccines for measles, mumps, and rubella were licensed and put into use. These viruses are all live attenuated (weakened) viruses. Since 1971, the

Parotid gland

A salivary gland (which makes saliva in the mouth) which is located at the jaw line just below the ear. The parotid gland can become swollen in children with mumps.

Rubella

A disease caused by the rubella virus. The disease is also called German measles or three-day measles.

In 25–50% of rubella infections there are no signs or symptoms of illness.

three vaccines have been combined in the MMR vaccine. This vaccine is now recommended to be given twice, first at age 12–15 months with a second at 4–6 years. One in 5 children can have a mild rash 1–2 weeks after the vaccine and some might have some swollen lymph nodes. One in 100 might have joint stiffness. Cases of encephalitis, or brain infection, have been reported; the frequency of this is < 1 per million children getting the vaccine. As discussed in a previous question, concern has been raised by some whether the vaccine has an association with the development of certain diseases such as autism, but scientific evidence does not confirm this (see question 15). The vaccines are very effective, with a reported > 99% protection from measles, 95% protection from rubella, and 90% protection from mumps after both doses (however, see answer to question 68).

Because the MMR is a live virus vaccine, there are more contraindications to receiving this vaccine when compared with other routine vaccines which are killed or inactivated. Children with minor illnesses such as a cold can safely receive the MMR, but the vaccine should usually be delayed if the illness is more severe. Children who have had a severe allergic reaction to a previous dose of the vaccine or who are known to be allergic to any of the vaccine components, including gelatin or the antibiotic neomycin, should not receive the vaccine. Children with a weakened immune system due to a medical condition or medicines (such as steroids) they are taking may have to delay immunization with the MMR. Also, children with low platelet counts or children who have recently received blood products may need to delay immunization. Finally, pregnancy is a contraindication for the vaccine, and teenage girls wanting to receive this vaccine should be urged to avoid getting pregnant within 4 weeks after getting the vaccine.

68. I heard about a mumps outbreak in people who had already received the vaccine? Why did that happen?

During a 9-month period in 2006, more than 5,000 cases of mumps were reported in the United States, which was the biggest outbreak in several decades. Other, smaller outbreaks have been reported. The strain of mumps virus that caused the outbreak was the same one which had caused a major outbreak in 56,000 people the previous year in the United Kingdom. In the larger United States outbreak in 2006, most people affected were young adults, including many college students. Air travel was shown to be an important factor in how rapidly the outbreak spread to many other states. Complications seen in this outbreak included 27 reports of orchitis (inflammation of the testes), 11 cases of meningitis, 4 cases of encephalitis, and the development of deafness in 4 patients.

In some prior outbreaks of mumps in the United States, one noted risk factor was that many people who became infected had not been up to date on immunization for mumps. However, public health officials are concerned that in this 2006 outbreak, the slight majority of people who developed mumps had received the two doses of MMR. Outbreaks in certain settings can occur despite high vaccination rates. Studies show that vaccine effectiveness with two mumps vaccinations is greater than the effectiveness following only one mumps vaccination. Studies are now ongoing to try to determine why this outbreak occurred. Specific questions to be answered are whether waning immunity was the major factor leading to this outbreak or whether a new, more effective type of mumps vaccine should be considered for use in the United States. Currently, the recommendation is still to receive the two doses of MMR, because this does provide protection against mumps in many, if not most, situations.

69. Can you take the three vaccines in the MMR separately?

The measles, mumps, and rubella vaccines are still produced and available as separate vaccines, but most physicians do not keep them in stock because they are not usually used. Since all three vaccines are recommended and can be given at the same time with one shot, most patients do not want separate vaccines. There are a few situations in which one vaccine may be desired separately. One example is in an outbreak situation for measles, where the recommendation may be to give the measles vaccine to infants 6 to 12 months old (before the usual time to give MMR) in order to protect infants who have a higher likelihood of being exposed to measles. Many providers will just give the MMR in that situation, but the separate vaccine for measles is available and could be used. In almost all situations, though, the three vaccines are given in the combined form.

In some live virus vaccines, such as the MMR, a very mild illness may develop due to the virus reproducing, but signs and symptoms of the regular disease should not develop.

70. I heard that the MMR is a live vaccine. Is a live virus vaccine more risky?

Since killed vaccines, toxoids, or subunit vaccines are not living and cannot reproduce in people, these vaccines cannot reproduce the infectious disease they are designed to protect against. Live virus vaccines are made from weakened forms of the virus which are designed to reproduce (replicate) in the vaccinated person but not give the disease. In some live virus vaccines, such as the MMR, a very mild illness may develop due to the virus reproducing, but signs and symptoms of the regular disease should not develop. Children who do not have a normal immune system, including children with an immune deficiency, advanced HIV infection, or types of cancers, should sometimes not receive these vaccines because there is some risk of getting a worse disease from the vaccine. Therefore, the vaccine is not considered risky for an otherwise healthy child, and it can and should be given as part of the usual vaccine schedule.

71. What is the varicella (chickenpox) vaccine?

Varicella zoster virus (VZV) is the virus which causes both chickenpox and shingles. A child who has never had chickenpox and never had the varicella vaccine is likely susceptible to infection with this virus. After a susceptible child is exposed to someone with chickenpox, the child will often become infected with the virus and develop chickenpox. Shingles, or zoster, is a recurrence of disease with the same virus. **Shingles**, which usually occurs later in life (if it ever occurs), presents with rash only in a small area of the skin. Before the vaccine was available, chickenpox was one of the most common childhood diseases. The peak age of this disease was in children younger than 10, and there were an average of 4 million cases per year in the United States. The peak season is in late winter to spring, but it can occur any time of year. Chickenpox is very contagious and spreads through the air from a cough, sneeze, or contact with the blisters in the rash.

Shingles

Also called zoster, this disease is a recurrence of disease with the virus that causes chickenpox (varicella).

Chickenpox often begins with fever, followed by a rash which comes in "crops" (at different times), is very pruritic (itches), and eventually spreads all over the body. Older children and adults often have a worse disease with a greater risk of scarring of the skin. The rash usually is crusted in a week. Usually chickenpox is mild, but complications can occur. The most common complication is infection of the blisters by bacteria. Less commonly, chickenpox can cause pneumonia and even brain infection. A baby born to a mother who has or is just getting chickenpox at the time of the baby's birth will have a more severe course than other children. Children with a weak immune system may also have more severe disease. There are medicines which can be used to treat chickenpox, but treatment must be started early in the illness to have any effect on the disease.

Varivax

The live virus vaccine used to prevent chickenpox (varicella).

The vaccine for chickenpox is called **Varivax**. It is a live, attenuated (weakened) virus vaccine which was licensed in 1995. Varivax is given at age 12–15 months and again at age 4–6 years. The vaccine is considered safe and is usually well-tolerated. Twenty percent of children will have a mild local reaction at the site of the shot and 10% will have some mild fever. In a small percentage of children, either a local rash or a more generalized rash will occur 1–3 weeks after the shot. If this vaccine-associated rash occurs, there are usually only a small number of pox lesions and they look more like small papules than the actual lesions of chickenpox. The vaccine is > 95% effective in preventing serious disease but only 70–90% effective in preventing any disease. The vaccine has been effective, and in some areas of the country the number of cases of chickenpox has dropped by 75–85%. However, chickenpox can occur in vaccinated children, and each year about 1% of people who receive the vaccine get chickenpox. The disease seen after immunization is usually much milder than typical chickenpox.

Because the varicella vaccine, like the MMR, is a live virus vaccine, many of the same precautions and contraindications discussed for the MMR are also true for this vaccine. As with most vaccines, children with minor illnesses such as a cold can safely receive the varicella vaccine, but the vaccine should usually be delayed if the illness is more severe. Children who have had a severe allergic reaction to a previous dose of the vaccine should not receive a second dose. Gelatin and the antibiotic neomycin are also components of the varicella vaccine; children known to be allergic to any of the vaccine components, including gelatin or neomycin, should not receive the vaccine. Children with a weakened immune system due to HIV infection, steroids, or medications to treat cancer may have to delay immunization with the MMR. Children who have recently received blood products may also need to delay immunization. As with the MMR, pregnancy is a contraindication for the varicella vaccine, and teenage girls wanting to receive this vaccine should be urged to avoid getting pregnant within 4 weeks after getting the vaccine.

Zostavax is a vaccine given to people to prevent the development of shingles. Currently it is used only in adults more than 60 years old and is not a childhood vaccine.

Zostavax
A vaccine given to people to prevent the development of shingles (zoster).

72. Chickenpox was common and not a severe illness. Why do we need a vaccine?

Usually chickenpox is a mild disease. However, before the use of the vaccine, approximately 50 children died every year from complications of chickenpox. If the chickenpox lesions become infected with bacteria, the resulting bacterial infection can become severe. The bacteria may cause infection only around the pox (skin lesion), but the infection can spread throughout the skin causing a cellulitis (skin infection) and into the blood causing infection in other sites in the body. One of the most severe complications is a type of skin infection called *necrotizing fasciitis*, which occurs in some infections with a type of bacteria called streptococcus. This is the same bacterium which causes "strep throat," but it is often called the "flesh-eating bacteria" by the news media when associated with this type of infection. A child with any type of secondary bacterial infection will usually require antibiotics and even hospitalization, depending on the severity of the infection.

Necrotizing fasciitis

A severe infection involving the skin and deeper tissues which is often caused by the same streptococcus bacterium that causes "strep throat."

Even if bacterial infections do not complicate the course of chickenpox, occasionally more severe disease with the virus itself can lead to other medical problems. Infection of the lung leading to a significant pneumonia is more common in adults than children. Infections of the brain are rare but can occur during or immediately following chickenpox. The use of aspirin in children with chickenpox was associated with a severe disease called Reye syndrome; educating parents to avoid the use of aspirin in children with chickenpox and other viral diseases has significantly decreased this complication.

Fortunately, chickenpox is usually a mild infection without severe complications. However, the illness often results in the child having to miss a week of school and parents to miss work to care for the child. Several studies have shown that use of the vaccine has led to fewer deaths, fewer hospitalizations, fewer visits to the doctor's office, and a decrease in overall expenses for chickenpox-related illnesses. Overall, the benefits of the vaccine have been shown to be significant.

73. I heard the varicella vaccine doesn't always work. Is this true?

The varicella vaccine is effective in preventing disease, but it is not perfect. One large study showed that the overall effectiveness of the vaccine was 87% for eight years after children received the vaccine. Severe disease due to chickenpox has decreased significantly with the use of the vaccine. However, some children still get "break-through" chickenpox. Most children previously immunized with the vaccine who have chickenpox have only a mild form of the disease. However, up to one third may have symptoms more like the typical infection. In addition, children with "break-through chickenpox" with the wild type virus are infectious to others, and have been the source of subsequent outbreaks in schools and daycares. In 2006, vaccine recommendations for the United States changed to include a second dose of the vaccine at age 4 to 6 years. The CDC and others are continuing to study the number of cases of chickenpox to make sure the current recommendations are the best for prevention of the disease.

Amy Lynn's comments:
We have seen kids who are exposed who had received the vaccine who did have chickenpox, but it was extremely light such as 5–6 "spots."

74. My first child received the varicella vaccine and afterwards had chickenpox. Does that happen often?

In 3–5% of children a local rash develops 1 to 3 weeks after giving the vaccine. In another 3–5 %, the rash is over more of the body. The skin lesions associated with the vaccine virus are often more maculopapular (raised spot without fluid) and differ in appearance from the true pox or vesicles of chickenpox. The number of pox is usually low and any associated signs or symptoms are usually mild if present at all. In some reported cases of chickenpox occurring shortly after the vaccine, the child was found to have been exposed to another child with chickenpox and the rash due to the real virus infection. This can happen during this time period because immunity against the virus would not have had enough time to develop if the child was exposed near the time of the immunization. Therefore, whether the rash is due to the vaccine or to actual chickenpox is sometimes difficult to discover. With the vaccine-associated rash, however, the illness is usually mild and without complication.

75. If my child gets a rash from the vaccine, is he contagious?

Children who get a vaccine-associated rash after immunization with the varicella vaccine usually have a small number of maculopapular lesions which often look different than true chickenpox. Children with definite vaccine-associated rash are considered to have a very low risk of transmitting virus. However, as stated in the previous question, sometimes real chickenpox may occur in children at this same time if they were exposed to someone with chickenpox, and it may be difficult to discover whether the rash is due to the vaccine or to actual chickenpox. Because true chickenpox is very contagious, most doctors advise parents that if the rash looks at all like chickenpox, they should treat their child as if they have chickenpox. Therefore, as one can often not be sure whether the rash is due to the vaccine strain or to regular chickenpox, it is best for the child with a rash during this time period to avoid contact with anyone at risk for chickenpox.

76. *What is the hepatitis A vaccine?*

Hepatitis A Virus is another cause of hepatitis. Unlike hepatitis B, which can cause a chronic hepatitis, hepatitis A causes disease that lasts several weeks. Before 2004, hepatitis A was the most frequently reported viral hepatitis in the United States. Before use of the vaccine, there were approximately 26,000 cases every year. Rates started to decline even before use of the vaccine. Historically, school-age children were one of the highest peaks for acquisition, but recently rates are highest in young adults. The virus is present in stool, and is spread by direct contact or from contaminated food or water.

Hepatitis A Virus (HAV)

A virus which can cause infection/inflammation of the liver.

Hepatitis A infection can produce disease of varying severity, and to some extent the severity is age-dependent. Children younger than 6 years of age often have no symptoms, and only 30% have yellow skin or eyes (jaundice). Older children and adults are more likely to have jaundice (> 70%), and may also have fever, nausea, vomiting, stomach pain, loss of appetite, and fatigue. Complications are unusual, although an average of 100 people per year die from hepatitis A-associated liver failure, sometimes because they had another type of liver disease in addition to this infection.

The hepatitis A virus vaccine was licensed in 1995 and became recommended for all children in the United States between ages of 12–23 months in 2005. The vaccine requires two doses, the second dose being given at least 6 months after the first. About half of children have a local reaction with < 10% having fever and fatigue. The vaccine has been shown to be from 94–100% effective in preventing hepatitis A in studies. The duration of protection is still being determined, but is thought to be at least 20 years.

Children with minor illnesses such as a cold can safely receive the Hepatitis A Vaccine. If your child has a more severe illness, the vaccine should usually be delayed until recovery from the illness. The vaccine should also not be given to any child who has experienced a life-threatening allergic reaction with a prior Hepatitis A Vaccine. As the vaccine contains alum and may contain the chemical 2-phenoxyethanol, if your child has a known allergy to these or other components in the vaccine, the vaccine should not be given. If your child is pregnant, the use of this vaccine should be discussed with their doctor. The Hepatitis A Vaccine is expected to be very safe when given during pregnancy, but the studies have yet to be reported to confirm this.

77. Once you have received the hepatitis B and hepatitis A vaccines, are you safe from hepatitis?

The viruses hepatitis A and hepatitis B cause a significant amount of the hepatitis we see in children. Unfortunately, however, there are many other viruses, and non-viral pathogens, which can affect the liver and cause hepatitis. **Hepatitis C Virus** is acquired similarly to hepatitis B, and also causes a chronic hepatitis which can lead to liver failure. Work on an effective vaccine for hepatitis C continues. Other types of viruses including enteroviruses, Epstein-Barr Virus (which causes "mono"), other herpes viruses, and other pathogens can cause hepatitis as part of their illness. In addition, hepatitis can be caused by certain medicines, alcohol, and other diseases. Therefore, use of the two hepatitis vaccines prevents two major causes of hepatitis but can never fully protect someone from getting disease of the liver.

Other types of viruses including enteroviruses, Epstein-Barr Virus (which causes "mono"), other herpes viruses, and other pathogens can cause hepatitis as part of their illness.

Hepatitis C Virus (HCV)

Another virus which can cause infection and/or inflammation of the liver.

PART SEVEN

Vaccines for School-Age Children and Teenagers

After age two will my child need more doses of some vaccines he has already received?

My child has a bad cut. How do I know if he needs another tetanus shot?

What is the meningococcal vaccine?

More . . .

78. After age two will my child need more doses of some vaccines he has already received?

Certain vaccines, for example rotavirus and *Haemophilus influenzae* type b vaccines, are needed for protection only in early childhood and are not recommended after age 2. Several vaccines already discussed are recommended for a booster dose between ages 4 and 6. These vaccines include the DTaP (diphtheria, tetanus, acellular pertussis), IPV (polio vaccine), Varicella Vaccine (for chickenpox), and the second MMR (measles, mumps, rubella). A tetanus booster should be given every ten years. This should be in the form of the Tdap (tetanus plus smaller doses of diphtheria and acellular pertussis) at age 11–12 years, and later the Td. In addition, children are currently advised to get an annual influenza immunization through age 18 (a new recommendation in 2008), and possibly beyond, depending upon the presence of certain risk factors. Catch-up immunization for other missed doses of vaccines may be given and, depending upon risk factors, additional doses of the pneumococcus vaccine may be given. These vaccines are all discussed in previous sections.

79. My child has a bad cut. How do I know if he needs another tetanus shot?

Most children 2 years of age and older have already had at least three doses of a tetanus vaccine. For minor wounds, children with at least three prior doses do not need a tetanus booster unless it has been 10 years or more since the last tetanus shot. If the wound is more than a minor wound, your child should get a tetanus booster if it has been more than five years since the last shot. If your child has had less than three tetanus shots, he should receive a tetanus booster for any type of wound. In addition, if the wound is serious, your doctor may give another shot which has tetanus antibody (**TIG, tetanus immune globulin**) to make sure your child is protected.

80. What is the meningococcal vaccine?

Neisseria meningitidis (**meningococcus**) is a type of bacteria which can cause life-threatening bloodstream infection and meningitis. It can cause infection in people of all ages. The highest rate of infection is in infants, with another peak of infection frequency in adolescents age 15–18, including freshmen in college living in dormitories. Infections are almost always severe and require hospitalization. These bacteria can be found in 5–10% of healthy people, in their nose and throat, and spread to others if there is close face to face contact or exposure to saliva from a person with the bacteria. The 5 major types of this bacterium are called Types A, B, C, Y, and W-135. Almost two thirds of cases in the United States are caused by types C and Y. Another third of total cases are caused by type B, but this type causes half of cases in infants.

Approximately 50% of serious meningococcal infections include meningitis, and one third have just infection in the bloodstream. Early symptoms include fever, chills, fatigue and a rash. In some people, the infection progresses so rapidly that death can occur in hours. Other symptoms include cough (due to pneumonia), conjunctivitis (red eyes), and signs of joint and heart effects. The overall death rate is 10–14% but it can be 25% in adolescents. Sequelae of severe infection can include brain damage, hearing loss, and amputation of fingers, toes, and limbs. Antibiotics can be used to treat the infection, but in severe disease they may not be used fast enough to prevent complications and death.

Tetanus immune globulin (TIG)

A preparation which contains antibody to tetanus. TIG can be given to anyone who is at risk of getting tetanus.

Neisseria meningitidis **(Meningococcus)**

A bacterium which can cause life-threatening bloodstream infection and meningitis.

Two vaccines to prevent this infection are licensed in the United States. In 2005, a conjugated meningococcal vaccine, MCV4, was licensed in the United States. Currently the vaccine is recommended for use in adolescents at 11–12 years of age, and to immunize any adolescent older than age 12 who is previously unimmunized with this vaccine. In addition, the vaccine is recommended for any child age 2 to 10 who is considered at high risk for meningococcal infection, including children with certain weakened immune systems or who lack a functioning spleen. The vaccine is being considered for use in all children age 2 years and above. A meningococcal polysaccharide vaccine (MPSV4) was licensed in 1981 and has been used for some time in high risk patients age 2 years and above. The newer conjugate vaccine (MCV4) is now preferred because it is thought to be better at eliminating carriage of the bacteria in the nose and providing long-term protection compared with the older vaccine. The "4" in the vaccine name means it works against 4 of the 5 types of bacteria. Unfortunately, neither vaccine is effective against Type B meningococcus.

These two meningococcal vaccines have an approximate 85% protection rate from infection with one of the four types in the vaccine. Both vaccines can have the side effect of localized pain at the site of the shot and headache, but both are mild and last only 1–2 days. Soon after the MCV4 vaccine was licensed in 2005, there was concern about several teenagers getting a nervous system disease called Guillain-Barre Syndrome. People at the FDA and CDC are continuing to monitor this but believe that the rate of the syndrome is the same as occurs without the vaccine, and they still recommend its use.

Children with minor illnesses such as a cold can safely receive either of the meningococcal vaccines. If your child has a more severe illness, the vaccine should usually be delayed until recovery from the illness. The vaccine should also not be given to any child who has experienced a life-threatening allergic reaction with a prior meningococcal vaccine or is known to be allergic to any of the vaccine components.

Abby's comments:

I am a senior in high school and will be heading off to college in a few months. I received the meningococcal vaccine a few months ago. I decided to get the vaccine due to the increased risk of contracting this type of meningitis in college and because it is recommended by colleges before you enter. It is a relatively painless way to help me be safer and healthier in college.

Mary Ellen's comments:

One of the most memorable cases of my career was the fulminant and fatal case of meningococcal meningitis in a young teen; it made a lasting impression on me. Yes, give the vaccine to all teenagers!

81. Does the meningococcal vaccine prevent meningitis?

Both types of meningococcal vaccine have a protection rate of about 85% against the four types of meningococcus in the vaccine. Meningococcus type B causes a significant amount of meningococcal meningitis in the United States, and it is not prevented by the vaccine.

Although the meningococcus is a significant cause of meningitis in children, there are many other types of bacteria and viruses which can cause meningitis. For

Both types of meningococcal vaccine have a protection rate of about 85% against the four types of meningococcus in the vaccine.

instance, meningitis caused by *Streptococcus pneumoniae* (pneumococcus) has been significantly decreased by use of the pneumococcal vaccine (see question 51). But there are many other causes of meningitis. Bacteria which can cause meningitis in children include *Streptococcus agalactiae* ("Group B Strep") and E. coli (both usually in young infants), *Haemophilus influenzae* (usually prevented by the Hib vaccine), Listeria, the bacterium causing tuberculosis, and others. Viruses are a common cause of meningitis and encephalitis. Viruses which can commonly affect the brain and its surrounding membranes include various types of enteroviruses, herpes, mosquito-borne viruses such as West Nile, and many others. None of these other infectious agents are impacted by the meningococcal vaccine; therefore meningitis is still a serious disease in children.

82. If my child is exposed to someone with meningitis, will she still need antibiotics to prevent her from getting it?

If you or your child has close personal contact with someone who is diagnosed with meningitis or severe infection due to meningococcus before they are treated, you or your child is considered to be at higher risk of getting the infection. For people with close contact, use of an antibiotic is recommended to decrease the risk of getting the disease. Several different antibiotics can be given and, depending on the antibiotic, it may be a single dose. As the meningococcal vaccine does not provide 100% protection against all types of meningococcus, an immunized person should still receive antibiotics. Your doctor can help decide who needs to receive antibiotics. For other causes of meningitis, antibiotics are usually not indicated for prevention.

83. Why are there two kinds of meningococcal vaccine? Which one should I request?

For many years, the only meningococcal vaccine available was the older polysaccharide vaccine. This was approved for use above age 2, and was used successfully for many situations. However, the newer conjugated vaccine seems to provide the same amount of protection against disease, helps get rid of meningococcus bacteria in the nose and throat, and protection seems to last longer. Therefore, the conjugate vaccine (MCV4) may replace much of the use of the older vaccine. In most situations, the newer vaccine should probably be used.

84. What is the HPV (papillomavirus) vaccine?

Human Papillomavirus, or **HPV**, is a common virus which causes various kinds of **warts**, including genital warts. There are more than 100 different types of HPV and some cause warts in different areas of the body. Cutaneous warts, or warts on the skin, are often detected in school age children. Skin warts, plantar warts, flat warts, and other kinds of warts are quite common in this age group. The warts can also be found on mucosal surfaces, including the nose and mouth. Genital warts are the most common sexually transmitted infection in the United States. Recent studies have shown that > 40% of sexually active adolescent females have genital HPV infection, and by age 50 more than 80% of women are HPV positive. Currently > 20 million men and women are infected with HPV.

Human Papillomavirus (HPV)

A common virus which causes various types of warts, including genital warts.

Warts

Common warts are small, often rough, lesions on the skin which are frequently seen on the hands or feet.

Most HPV infections are asymptomatic, and although the infection clears spontaneously, it may take a couple of years to do so. Anogenital warts present on the penis, scrotum, anal or perianal area in men and on the vulva, perianal area and, less commonly, cervix or in the vagina in women. Usually they are painless, although they can cause itching, burning, pain, and bleeding. The optimal treatment of warts is not known, but various topical therapies and local injections of antiviral agents have been attempted if treatment is deemed necessary. The most significant complication of HPV is the association of the virus with **dysplastic lesions**. HPV causes >99% of **cervical cancers** and can also cause vulvar, anal, and penile cancers. Certain types of HPV are high risk for causing cancer. Types 16 and 18 cause 70% of cervical cancers, but types 31, 45, and at least 14 other types are also considered high risk.

In 2006, the FDA licensed **Gardasil**, the first HPV Vaccine. This vaccine is a quadrivalent vaccine containing material from four types: Types 16, 18, 6, and 11. The first two types are high risk for causing cervical cancer and the latter two types cause the majority of genital warts as well as most warts which have spread to the respiratory tract. The vaccine induces a good immune response and is considered very safe. The vaccine is recommended for routine immunization for adolescent girls at age 11–12; it is recommended for older adolescent females if not already immunized. The schedule for giving the vaccine is a three-dose series, with the second dose 2 months after the first and the third dose 4 months after the second. The vaccine is given as a shot in the shoulder muscle.

Children with minor illnesses can safely receive the HPV Vaccine, but the vaccine should usually be delayed until after recovery if the illness is more severe. The

Dysplastic lesions

Areas of skin or mucosa (e.g., in an area on the cervix seen on a pap smear) which show abnormal development or growth of cells or tissues.

Cervical cancers

Cancer of the cervix (lower part of the uterus) or areas around the cervix. Cervical cancer can present with bleeding but often has no symptoms until the cancer is advanced.

Gardasil

The first HPV vaccine approved in the United States.

vaccine should also not be given to any child who has experienced a life-threatening allergic reaction with a prior HPV Vaccine, or who is allergic to any components of the vaccine, including yeast. Currently pregnancy is considered a contraindication for the HPV vaccine.

85. What types of cancer does this vaccine prevent?

The major cancer caused by certain types of HPV is cervical cancer. HPV causes almost all cervical cancers and precancerous lesions of the cervix. It also causes a large proportion of cancer and precancerous lesions in other anogenital sites in both men and women, including vulvar cancer, anal cancers, and penile cancers. Cervical cancer is diagnosed in almost 10,000 United States women every year and has recently caused about 3,700 deaths per year. Approximately 70% of the cervical cancers are caused by HPV Types 16 and 18, which are in the currently approved vaccine.

HPV causes almost all cervical cancers and precancerous lesions of the cervix.

86. Why has this vaccine caused a lot of controversy?

Gardasil, the only currently available HPV Vaccine, was licensed by the FDA in early 2006. Later the same month, the CDC Advisory Committee on Immunization Practices (ACIP) voted to recommend routine immunization with HPV Vaccine for all girls 11–12 years of age. The vaccine was quickly promoted and recommended for routine use. In early 2007, the governor of the state of Texas issued a mandate for all girls in the state of Texas who were 11–12 years of age to have the vaccine prior to entering the sixth grade. This mandate, and other efforts to require the use of this vaccine, met with significant controversy.

Sexually-transmitted disease (STD)

Any infection or disease which is transmitted to someone else by unprotected sex.

Most of the controversy was not about the effectiveness of the vaccine, but instead about the fact that a relatively new vaccine against a **sexually-transmitted disease (STD)** was going to be mandated for young girls. Some parents did not want to give a vaccine against an STD to a pre-teen girl, while others did not want their child to receive the vaccine at any age, because many believed their daughters were not or would not be at risk for an STD. Since there were still questions about the duration of protection afforded by the vaccine, there were concerns that giving the vaccine too early would risk decreased protection at a time when protection was needed at older ages. There was also concern by some that any vaccine against an STD might increase promiscuity because it could foster the belief that the girl was safe against all STDs. Opponents believed efforts should be made toward trying to prevent premarital sex instead of using a vaccine on the assumption that it would occur. Even some vaccine experts were not in favor of the rapid institution of mandates for the vaccine, believing that such mandates without prior sufficient education for the public on the use and benefits of the vaccine would lead to mistrust of the vaccine.

Although these mandates and the controversy which followed did lead to some backlash against use of the vaccine, education of the public about the vaccine and its benefits has led to increasing acceptance and use of the vaccine.

Abby's comments:

I think most girls that get this vaccine understand that it doesn't protect them against all STDs. Considering it protects you from risk of some types of cancers when you're older, it seems like a great idea. But I'm not sure if it should be mandatory.

87. My daughter is not having sex yet. Why does she need this vaccine?

The HPV vaccine has been recommended to be given to girls at 11–12 years of age because the vaccine is most effective when given prior to sexual activity and exposure to HPV. The vaccine has been shown to be less effective in preventing precancerous lesions in women already exposed to HPV types 16 and 18. The vaccine has little or no beneficial effect if infection with the HPV types in the vaccine has already occurred. These studies, therefore, support giving the vaccine at an age prior to onset of sexual activity.

While many parents do not believe children need an STD vaccine at an early age, unfortunately, current statistics support such a need for many young girls. For example, results of the CDC 2005 Youth Risk Behavior Survey were tabulated and showed that 47% of high school students in the survey had sexual intercourse, and 34% of sexually active students did not use a condom the last time they had sexual intercourse. In the ninth grade, 34% of students reported having had sexual intercourse. Therefore, many young girls are in fact at risk of HPV acquisition. It is important to note that even if a child is abstinent until marriage, there is no guarantee that her partner practiced abstinence. CDC reports have documented that >14% of women age 18–25 with only one lifetime sexual partner had HPV. The decision to use the vaccine is yours, but with risk of HPV acquisition being high, the benefits of the vaccine are significant.

Abby's comments:

I have received all three shots of Gardasil. I am not sexually active but I believe it's better to get it before you come upon a situation where you are at risk. I know a lot of people at my school who are sexually active and many of their parents don't know.

88. Should teenage boys get the HPV vaccine?

Human papillomavirus is probably as common, if not more common, in men as it is in women. Recent studies have shown that teenage males have a high prevalence of genital HPV, and are therefore infectious to females. HPV is not as easily diagnosed in males as in females. Men become infected with HPV like women, by vaginal or anal sex. Also like women, there are no symptoms with infection unless the HPV type can cause genital warts. In men, genital warts can form around the anus, penis, scrotum, or groin.

HPV-associated cancer in men is much less than that seen in women. However, the American Cancer Society estimates that >1,250 men will be diagnosed with penile and other types of genital cancers and >2,000 with anal cancers in 2008. A growing number of head and neck cancers are also associated with HPV. Perhaps most important, though, is that HPV-infected males can pass the infection to their partners, and prevention of infection in males would decrease HPV infection and HPV-related cancers in women.

Males have been included in HPV vaccine studies to prove the vaccine is safe and creates an immune response. Studies are still underway to see whether the vaccine protects males from HPV infections and related conditions and whether it can prevent passing the virus to their partners, which should in turn reduce cervical cancer. At the current time, there is no HPV vaccine licensed for use in males. Within the next couple of years, the FDA will likely consider licensing HPV vaccines for use in boys and men, and decisions will need to be made regarding recommendations for its use in teenage boys.

Abby's comments:

Even though men can't get cervical cancer, boys should still get the shot so that their girlfriends or wives won't get cervical cancer. It's a small price for them to pay to get a few shots to prevent cancer in women and perhaps themselves.

89. I heard there is another HPV vaccine coming out. Which one should we use?

A second HPV vaccine will likely be licensed for use in adolescent girls in late 2008 or 2009. This vaccine, called **Cervarix**, is effective against HPV Types 16 and 18, similar to Gardasil. The design of this vaccine differs from the Gardasil vaccine. The company which produces Cervarix states it may provide protection against other types of the virus and may provide protection for a longer period of time, but this is still being evaluated. Further details and recommendations regarding this vaccine will be available after licensure and your child's doctor can assist with recommendations regarding which vaccine would be most beneficial to use.

Cervarix

A second HPV vaccine which is expected to be licensed for use in adolescent girls in late 2008 or 2009.

PART EIGHT

Special Situations and Special Vaccines

Are there any other vaccines my child might have to receive?

We are adopting a child from a foreign country. What vaccines will she need?

Is there a vaccine for TB (tuberculosis)?

More . . .

90. Are there any other vaccines my child might have to receive?

There are a few special situations in which a vaccine not recommended for all children might be indicated or recommended for your child. Such situations may involve a known exposure to a certain infectious agent (e.g., exposure to rabies) or an increased possibility of exposure to a specific disease due to illness in a family member or travel. If you have concerns about the possible need for further immunizations due to known or anticipated exposures, contact your physician or health department to check on current recommendations for additional vaccines.

91. We are adopting a child from a foreign country. What vaccines will she need?

Soon after arrival to the United States, a healthcare provider should evaluate internationally adopted children for the presence of acute and chronic infections, as well as to determine their status regarding their need for immunizations.

Many couples and individuals are adopting children from foreign countries. The recent estimates are that more than 20,000 internationally adopted children arrive in the United States every year. The majority of children are being adopted from China, Russia, Guatemala, the Ukraine, and a short list of other countries. Many of these countries have a higher incidence of many infectious diseases, including some which are rarely encountered in the United States. In addition, many adopted children have been living in suboptimal circumstances. For some children, malnutrition, emotional stress, and suboptimal medical care have adversely affected their immune systems and their general health.

Soon after arrival to the United States, a healthcare provider should evaluate internationally adopted children for the presence of acute and chronic infections, as well as to determine their status regarding their need for immunizations. Usually children are tested for syphilis, HIV, hepatitis B, and perhaps hepatitis C, tuberculosis, and intestinal parasites. If immunization records are available, the provider will need to review the records to help decide which vaccines need to be given. Some vaccines which are considered part of the routine immunization schedule in the United States are not available in some countries (examples may include the varicella vaccine and conjugated vaccines for pneumococcus and *Haemophilus influenzae*). These vaccines will need to be administered dependent upon the age of the child. In some settings, reliability of the records and/or the effectiveness of vaccines previously given are in question. Some doctors choose to check the child's blood for evidence of a response to certain vaccines to help make the decision as to whether some need to be repeated. If no immunization records exist, which may be the case for some children, the doctor may have to assume that no vaccines have been given and proceed from the beginning with immunizations for the child. If this needs to be done, differing schedules exist for the administration of vaccines, dependent upon the age of the child.

92. Is there a vaccine for TB (tuberculosis)?

Tuberculosis (TB) is the disease caused by the bacterium *Mycobacterium tuberculosis*. Most people think of TB as a disease of the lungs, but many parts of the body can be affected. The World Health Organization estimates that there are more than 8 million new cases of TB and 1.6 million deaths in the world due to TB every year. In 2006, almost 14,000 new cases were reported in the United States, with 6% of those in children. In the United States, people who live in large cities, have

Tuberculosis (TB)
The disease caused by the bacterium *Mycobacterium tuberculosis*.

Most people think of TB as a disease of the lungs, but many parts of the body can be affected.

low incomes, are non-whites or are foreign-born are at a higher risk of getting TB. The bacteria spread through the air from one person to another. People can become infected when someone with active TB lung disease coughs and the bacteria are breathed in by others. Most people who become infected do not get sick, but the bacteria stay in the body causing a latent infection. People with latent TB are not ill and cannot spread the infection to others. However, at any time the bacteria can reactivate, start causing disease, and make that person infectious to others. You can be tested for TB by getting a skin test, which will usually be positive if you are infected with TB. If you have lung disease or other types of disease, your doctor can check your sputum for TB. Antibiotics are available to treat the disease, but effective treatment requires many months of antibiotics and some bacteria are becoming more resistant to the drugs.

Most infections in children are asymptomatic. Infants and older teenagers are more likely to progress to the active disease compared with children of other ages and adults. The first symptoms and signs of active TB are fever, cough, weight loss, and night sweats. A chest x-ray can show a pneumonia, a cavity (less likely in children), or large lymph nodes in the chest. TB can cause a meningitis or infection in the brain, and infants and young children are more likely than adults to get this complication. In addition to the lung and brain, TB can infect the lymph nodes, bone, skin, ear, and other parts of the body.

The first symptoms and signs of active TB are fever, cough, weight loss, and night sweats.

BCG (Bacille Calmette-Guérin):

A vaccine for tuberculosis (TB) which is given to children in many countries with high rates of TB to try to prevent the disease in children.

BCG, or **Bacille Calmette-Guérin**, is a vaccine for TB which is given to children in many countries with high rates of TB to try to prevent the disease. Two TB vaccines are available in the United States and many others are used in other countries. The BCG vaccine gives about 80% protection against certain types of disease (such as infection in the brain), but overall protection is about 50%. BCG is not recommended for children in the United States, due in part to the lower risk of infection in this country. There are only a few special circumstances where it might be used in the United States. Doctors might recommend use of BCG vaccine for a child who cannot be separated from a person who has active or more resistant tuberculosis. The vaccine can cause a local reaction such as a small abscess under the skin or large lymph nodes in 1–2% of people. Rarely, BCG vaccine causes a bone infection or other serious infections. Scientists are trying to make a better vaccine against TB, and possibly in the future a vaccine for TB will be used in the United States.

Anyone with burns, skin infections, or any type of immune deficiency such as HIV should not receive the BCG vaccine. In addition, anyone taking medicines which weaken the immune system, such as high doses of steroids, should not get the vaccine.

93. Is there a vaccine for Lyme disease?

Lyme disease is caused by a microorganism called *Borrelia burgdorferi*. The disease takes its name from Lyme, Connecticut, where the full spectrum of illness was first described in 1975. This germ normally lives in mice, squirrels, and other small animals, and is passed on to people by the bite of an infected blacklegged tick (e.g., deer tick). The results of infection can include a characteristic rash and other symptoms, with occasional more severe complications of untreated disease. In 2006, almost 20,000 cases of Lyme disease were reported in the United States, with the majority of the cases reported in the New England states and the upper Midwest. Lyme disease can occur at any age but is most common in

Lyme disease

An infectious disease caused by a microorganism called *Borrelia burgdorferi.*

children ages 5 to 19 and in boys more than girls. The peak season for infection is summer. Diagnosis of the disease is usually by recognition of the rash and other symptoms, but blood can be sent for Lyme testing in later stages of the disease. Most cases can be successfully treated with antibiotics, especially if treatment is started early in the disease.

The first sign of Lyme disease is usually a characteristic circular red rash called erythema migrans. This rash begins as early as a few days to as late as a month after the tick bite. Fatigue, fever, chills, headache, muscle and joint pains, and swollen lymph nodes can occur with the rash. If untreated, some people with Lyme disease can have later complications with effects on the joints, the brain and nervous system, and the heart.

LYMErix

A vaccine against Lyme disease approved for use in the United States in 1998, but soon taken off the market.

LYMErix, a vaccine against Lyme disease, was approved for use in the United States in 1998. The vaccine contains a protein from the outer surface of the germ. Initial clinical studies showed the vaccine to be safe and close to 80% effective after three doses. However, the vaccine was taken off the market by the manufacturer in 2002. The reason cited by the company was poor demand for the vaccine. Some Lyme disease patients and advocacy groups believe the reason was more complex; some had concerns that the vaccine was less effective in preventing Lyme disease, had only a short duration of protection, and possibly caused more side effects than expected, especially in people who had previously had Lyme disease. Efforts to find a better vaccine for Lyme disease continue, but currently no vaccine is available.

94. My child loves animals. Does she need a rabies vaccine?

Infection with **rabies** virus causes a severe disease of the brain and nervous system that is almost always fatal. Fortunately, rabies virus infection in humans in the United States is rare, recently averaging only 2–3 cases per year. In 2006, almost 7,000 cases of rabies were reported in animals in the United States. More than 90% of animal cases are in wild animals, with infections in raccoon, bats, and skunks being most commonly reported. In domesticated animals, rabid cats are most frequently reported, followed by cattle and dogs. Rabies is usually acquired from the bite of an infected animal, and most recent cases in the United States are due to bites from infected bats. Rabies is confirmed in animals by testing samples of brain tissue for the virus. In people, samples of blood, saliva, cerebrospinal fluid, and a biopsy of skin from the hairline at the back of the neck can be collected for rabies tests. Treatment for rabies often consists of giving supportive care. One child who had rabies in the United States in 2004 was treated with antiviral drugs and survived, although most people die from rabies despite use of these medicines.

The signs and symptoms of rabies are noticed an average of 4 to 6 weeks after the bite, but the time can be as soon as a week to as long as several years. Early symptoms are non-specific and can include fever, headache, and fatigue. Later signs of rabies may include anxiety, confusion, agitation, seizures, and increase in salivation with problems swallowing. Death occurs days after these latter symptoms begin.

Rabies

A severe disease of the brain and nervous system caused by rabies virus infection. The disease is almost always fatal. Bites from an infected bat currently cause most of the human cases of rabies in the United States.

There are two brands of rabies virus vaccine, and both are killed virus preparations. If your child does have an exposure to rabies, she should receive a dose of rabies vaccine plus a preparation of rabies antibody, both given as a shot, soon after the exposure. The rabies vaccine series should be completed by giving another dose of the vaccine on days 3, 7, 14, and 28 days after the first dose of vaccine. Rabies vaccine is given before exposures only to select groups of people who may have a higher risk of exposure to rabid animals, such as veterinarians or animal handlers. Children are not considered at risk simply due to routine animal exposures. Rabies vaccine should be given to children following possible rabies exposures, such as bites from certain wild animals or domesticated animals who lack or have unknown rabies vaccine history. If a bat is found in the room where a young child has been sleeping, rabies vaccine should be started. Your child's physician or the local health department can provide further advice on whether rabies vaccine should be given dependent upon the exposure. There are significantly fewer side effects with current rabies vaccines compared with vaccines used in the past. Both of the current vaccines are well tolerated, with the most common reaction being a mild skin reaction at the site of the injection, as occurs with many vaccines.

The seriousness of rabies and the benefits of vaccine use in prevention of the disease create a situation where there are few true contraindications to use of the vaccine for true rabies exposures. If a severe allergic reaction does occur, it may be advisable to switch to the other brand of vaccine not initially used.

95. *Is there a vaccine that prevents HIV/AIDS?*

HIV, which stands for Human Immunodeficiency Virus, is the virus that causes AIDS. The worldwide statistics on HIV infection are staggering. As of 2008, it was estimated that 65 million people have been infected with HIV, with 40 million people currently living with HIV/**AIDS** worldwide, and more than 2 million in this number being children younger than age 15. In 2006, there were approximately 4.3 million new infections and 2.9 million deaths due to HIV. Worldwide, more than 4 million children have died from AIDS. Current studies show that the southern United States has the majority of newly diagnosed HIV infections (46%; adults and children) in the United States, and nationwide many new infections are in adolescents. HIV is found in blood and semen or vaginal fluid in an infected person. Transmission to others does not occur with everyday activities such as kissing, hugging, and sharing utensils. But virus can be transmitted by having unprotected sex (anal, vaginal, or oral) with someone infected with HIV, sharing needles and syringes with someone infected with HIV, or being exposed (fetus or infant) to HIV before or during birth or through breast feeding. All donated blood in the United States is screened for HIV, and the current risk of transmission in a blood transfusion is extremely low.

HIV acts in the body mainly by attacking certain cells in the immune system. Since the immune system helps to protect our body from many types of infections, people with advanced HIV disease can get a variety of infections and other illnesses, many of which are not usually seen in healthy people. AIDS, which stands for acquired immunodeficiency syndrome, is the final stage of HIV infection. People differ tremendously in

Human Immunodeficiency Virus (HIV)

The virus that causes AIDS. Although significant efforts have been made to find an effective vaccine, there is currently no vaccine available to prevent infection with HIV.

As of 2008, it was estimated that 65 million people have been infected with HIV, with 40 million people currently living with HIV/AIDS worldwide, and more than 2 million in this number being children younger than age 15.

AIDS

Acquired Immunodeficiency Syndrome, the final stage of HIV infection caused by virus-induced destruction of the immune system.

the course of HIV infection. It can take many years for some people infected with HIV to progress to AIDS, even without treatment, while others seem to progress to AIDS more rapidly. There are effective drugs available to treat HIV. These drugs, when used correctly, can help to suppress the virus and keep people healthy, but the drugs cannot cure HIV. A major problem with treatment is the development of resistance of the virus to the drugs being used, which may lead to fewer treatment options (and sometimes no treatment options) for that person in the future.

Scientists have been working to find a vaccine to prevent HIV for more than 25 years. Research efforts are continuing, but to date there are no effective vaccines to prevent HIV infection. Vaccine candidates are also being studied to see if a type of vaccine can be developed which would boost the immune system of a person who already has HIV, thereby helping that person fight the virus. HIV vaccine efforts suffered a setback in late 2007. Two vaccine trials using one of the top vaccine candidates showed that not only was the vaccine not effective, it may have even increased some people's risk of getting HIV. These vaccines did not contain any virus capable of causing HIV infection, but scientists are trying to understand how vaccine effects on the immune system may have increased the susceptibility to infection in some people. At the time of the writing of this book, scientists are regrouping to reevaluate the best strategies for development of an effective HIV vaccine. Development of a successful HIV vaccine is of great importance worldwide, and hopefully there will be success with other strategies.

96. If my child travels outside the United States, does he need additional vaccines?

Travel outside of the United States often increases the risk of certain infections for a child. Vaccine recommendations, and recommendations for other medications, vary depending upon the countries to be visited and activities in that country. Routine immunizations recommended in the United States should be up-to-date in the child because many of these vaccine-preventable diseases are present in greater frequency in other countries. Occasionally, the vaccine schedule may even be "moved up" to provide earlier protection dependent upon the age of the child. Additional vaccines may be recommended for travel to certain areas. Examples of vaccines not recommended for United States children, but occasionally recommended for travelers, include vaccines for yellow fever, Japanese Encephalitis Virus, and typhoid fever. A few countries may require vaccines such as yellow fever for entry into some countries in South America or Africa.

Yellow Fever virus is transmitted to humans through the bite of infected mosquitoes. The virus is maintained in nature by transmission among nonhuman primates. The disease occurs only in sub-Saharan Africa and the tropics of South America. The disease yellow fever ranges in severity from a more benign illness similar to influenza (the flu) to severe hepatitis and hemorrhagic fever. The illness can be quite severe, and in Africa the mortality rate is about 20%, with infants and children at greatest risk of severe disease.

Yellow Fever

A disease caused by Yellow Fever virus. This virus is found mainly in parts of Africa and South America and is transmitted to humans via infected mosquitoes.

The yellow fever vaccine is a live, attenuated (weakened) vaccine given in a single dose. It is recommended for infants older than 9 months through adults who will be traveling in an area at risk for yellow fever exposure. Infants younger than 9 months may be considered for immunization with the vaccine, but the risks and benefits should be discussed with your doctor. Although the vaccine is usually tolerated well, up to 25% of people getting the vaccine may have a mild reaction which can include headache, muscle aches, and low-grade fever. Severe reactions including encephalitis (infection of the brain) and other severe reactions have been reported, but are rare. The vaccine is a live vaccine which is prepared in eggs, and possible contraindications for vaccine use in your child should be discussed with your child's doctor.

Japanese Encephalitis

A disease caused by the Japanese Encephalitis virus. It is prevalent in areas of Asia and Australia, and is transmitted to humans via the bite of infected mosquitoes. Infection with the virus can cause encephalitis. A killed vaccine is available for travelers to areas where the virus is commonly found.

Japanese Encephalitis virus is also transmitted to people through the bite of an infected mosquito. It occurs throughout much of Southeast Asia, as far west as Pakistan and India, as far east as Eastern Russia and Japan, and as far south as Australia. The disease caused by infection with this virus is the most common cause of encephalitis (brain infection) in that part of the world. Up to 50,000 cases and 15,000 deaths are reported to the World Health Organization every year, and children are at greatest risk of infection. Most infections are asymptomatic, with only one in 250 people infected with the virus developing any symptoms of the disease. Milder symptoms such as fever with headache are more likely seen in adults, but overall encephalitis is the most common disease. There is no specific treatment for this virus infection.

The Japanese Encephalitis Virus Vaccine approved in the United States is a killed vaccine produced in the brains of mice, but a newer killed vaccine produced in the laboratory in other types of cells should soon be available. The vaccine is recommended for people traveling for an extended period (> 30 days) to areas at risk of virus exposure, and occasionally to those traveling for a shorter stay if the area is experiencing an epidemic. The usual vaccine series is in three doses, given at days 0, 7, and 30. The vaccine can be used in children above the age of one year, although the dosage given to children 1–3 years of age is half the adult dose. Reactions to the vaccine such as generalized itching and swelling can occur in 0.3% of people receiving the vaccine. Contraindications for the vaccine can be discussed with your child's doctor.

Typhoid fever is an acute, life-threatening illness with fever caused by the bacterium *Salmonella enterica* serotype Typhi, or sometimes called *Salmonella typhi*. There are many similar strains of salmonella in the United States which are often associated with bloody diarrhea, but not usually the type of severe illness seen in typhoid fever. This disease occurs in an estimated 22 million people with 200,000 deaths worldwide. In the United States, an average of 400 cases of typhoid are reported every year, and most people diagnosed with typhoid had recently traveled outside the United States. Areas at risk for acquiring typhoid fever include South Asia and developing countries in Asia, Africa, Central and South America and the Caribbean. Salmonella typhi is found only in humans (not in animals), but can be spread via food and water contaminated by infected people. People with a chronic infection can transmit infection to many other people, as is well illustrated by a famous Irish Immigrant in New York City in the early 1900s, "Typhoid Mary." This woman had an asymptomatic infection and, unfortunately, became famous for the number of people she infected in her daily duties as a

Typhoid fever

An acute, life-threatening illness with fever caused by the bacteria *Salmonella typhi*. Two types of vaccines are available for use for the prevention of infection with this bacterium.

In the United States, an average of 400 cases of typhoid are reported every year, and most people diagnosed with typhoid had recently traveled outside the United States.

cook. Acute infection with typhoid consists of mainly high fever (103–104) with headache, fatigue, enlarged spleen, and a distinctive rash. Mild and even asymptomatic infections can occur. Antibiotics are given for treatment of the infection.

Two typhoid vaccines are available in the United States, a live attenuated (weakened) vaccine taken by mouth and a subunit vaccine which contains part of the bacterial capsule to be taken by shot. Both vaccines protect 50–80% of people immunized. The oral vaccine (given by mouth) is given in four doses, each separated by two days. Only one dose of the shot is required for the first immunization. Booster doses of both vaccines are required. Children younger than age 6 (years) should not receive the oral vaccine, and children less than age 2 should not receive either vaccine. Both vaccines are fairly well tolerated, but some children taking the oral vaccine may have mild abdominal discomfort, nausea, vomiting, fever, headache and rash, while fever, headache, and a local skin reaction are seen with the vaccine given by shot. Contraindications for the vaccine can be discussed with your child's doctor.

Additional vaccines and medications may be recommended for children traveling out of the country, and your child's doctor can assist in determining which vaccines and medicines are needed or recommended. Ideally your child should see the doctor well in advance (at least 4–6 weeks) prior to travel in order to begin any vaccine series needed for travel. Many vaccines do not create sufficient immunity in a short period of time and immunity should be optimum at the beginning of the trip. Your doctor will be able to provide recommendations for vaccines needed for travel if provided with the travel itinerary, although the information should be given to the doctor in advance of your child's visit, if possible, to allow the doctor's office enough time to obtain the needed vaccines. A useful website for up-to-date travel information is the CDC Travel Health website at *www.cdc.gov/travel*. The CDC also publishes a book with the same information (the "Yellow Book") which can usually be found in a public library or ordered from the CDC.

97. I have heard people talk about vaccines for smallpox and anthrax. Are those vaccines for children?

During the past few years, there has been increased talk of the risk of bioterrorism and whether people in the United States should receive vaccines for some commonly discussed agents of bioterrorism. Two common germs discussed are smallpox and anthrax.

Smallpox was a disease well-known for its presentation with high fever, spots or lesions in the mouth, and then the appearance of a rash with classic "pox" lesions. The rash was often extensive, lasted a couple of weeks, and often caused scarring. The disease was very contagious, often severe, and sometimes fatal.

Fortunately, smallpox is now also known for being the first virus infection which was successfully eradicated from the world because of the use of vaccines. As it was eradicated, the decision was made to stop routine vaccination for smallpox many years ago. The only samples of the virus are maintained in a few laboratories, but there has been concern that terrorists may acquire the virus and try to start another epidemic. A new vaccine for smallpox, ACAM2000, was licensed in 2007. The vaccine consists of live vaccinia virus (virus similar to smallpox which does not give the same disease). As of March 2008, this vaccine is the smallpox vaccine being given to selected personnel in the military, state public health preparedness programs, and laboratory personnel. It is currently not recommended for the general public.

Unlike the smallpox virus, the bacterium *Bacillus anthracis*, which causes **anthrax**, has already been used in attempted bioterrorism activities. The bacteria causing anthrax are found in soils around the world. These bacteria can produce spores which can remain in the soil for decades. Various animals can get anthrax, and people coming in contact with infected animals or contaminated animal products can get the disease. Most naturally acquired infections in people are infections of skin, but more severe infections of the lungs or stomach and intestines can occur. The pneumonia is the worst form of the disease. Antibiotics can be used to treat the infection, but must be given early to be effective in the most severe forms of disease.

Bacillus anthracis is one of the most likely germs to be used as a biological weapon because the spores are very stable, the spores can infect the respiratory route and lungs, and lung disease with anthrax has a high mortality rate. A vaccine is available, but it must be given in an initial series of six doses followed by a booster vaccine every year. The anthrax vaccine is not recommended for the general public at this time, but is used in the military and other populations considered high risk.

There are many other infectious agents which scientists and public health officials believe might be used for bioterrorism. Efforts continue to create effective treatments for the diseases associated with these agents, as well as to create safer and more effective vaccines in case these threats of bioterrorism materialize.

Anthrax

The disease caused by infection with the bacterium *Bacillus anthracis*.

98. *What new vaccines might be available soon?*

Numerous vaccines are currently in development and may be approved for use in the near future. Some vaccines currently being evaluated are newer versions of older vaccines already in use for children. The goal is to see if vaccines with greater safety and effectiveness can be designed. Vaccines against common childhood infections, such as respiratory syncytial virus (RSV; a cause of pneumonia and respiratory infections) and herpes simplex virus (HSV; cause of herpes in the mouth and genital herpes) are in various stages of development. Work is being done on vaccines for infectious agents that cause significant chronic disease throughout the United States, such as Hepatitis C Virus (a significant cause of chronic hepatitis), as well as for germs associated with recent "emerging infections" such as the West Nile Virus, which can cause brain infections such as encephalitis and meningitis. Research is underway to create effective vaccines for diseases such as malaria and dengue fever, which are so important worldwide. Vaccines for such "tropical diseases" would probably not be used routinely in the United States, unless you and your child were traveling to a foreign country where the disease was common. However, there has been concern that changes in climate may lead to an increase of naturally occurring tropical diseases in our southern states, and such vaccines may need to be considered for the United States in the future.

Another exciting development in vaccine technology is the creation of new ways to give vaccines. Several "needle-less" techniques are being developed, including the use of a skin patch and other methods, for eventual use in giving routine vaccines without a "shot." Even edible vaccines, such as potatoes and bananas in which a vaccine strain of bacteria or virus is introduced, may be a method for giving children some of their routine vaccines. These technologies are probably at least several years away, but give hope for even safer, less painful means of immunizing our children, and ourselves, in the future.

PART NINE

Recommended Resources for Information

I get confused with different opinions on vaccines.
How can I get the truth?

Where can I find more information on
childhood immunizations?

More . . .

99. I get confused with different opinions on vaccines. How can I get the truth?

A large amount of vaccine information is available on the internet, in books, and in radio or television talk shows. You may note that the information may often be contradictory, and it is difficult to know what sources to trust. Information against vaccine use and information for vaccine use can be very flawed, and one always needs to consider the source of the information. This is especially true for web-based information. The website should state who is responsible for the website, and information should not be slanted toward the website's sponsor or funding source. If medical or scientific information is given, one should ask whether credible scientific or medical experts review the information, if they revise and update the information, and if they document the exact source of the medical claims. Often the purpose of the website is related to a specific product, and one should be skeptical in this setting. Although accurate information is sometimes given on someone's private website or blog or the website of a small, unknown organization, this is generally less reliable. Likewise, the website of a pharmaceutical company which produces the specific vaccine is not likely to present in-depth information on possible adverse effects. The most accurate sources of information are well-respected medical or scientific organizations including the CDC (Center for Disease Control), AAP (American Academy of Pediatrics), WHO (World Health Organization), etc. The best advice is to discuss the information with a doctor or health care professional you trust.

Amy Lynn's comments:

It is important to have a pediatrician that you trust to pro-vide correct information. If I have a question about some-thing, I ask, "If this was your child, what would you do?" There is also a lot of information available on the internet about different vaccines, but you have to be careful to check the source for dependability.

100. Where can I find more information on childhood immunizations?

The following Appendix provides a list of resources for parents relating to childhood immunizations. The sections are divided into different types of educational media, including Internet websites, books, publications from the CDC and other government agencies, videos, and other educational formats. As discussed in the answer to question 99, there is, unfortunately, a great amount of information in all educational formats which provides very different information about vaccines. It is a challenge to try to determine which information is accurate and up-to-date. Hopefully the use of these resources, coupled with use of this book, will help guide parents in their search for accurate information to help them make decisions regarding childhood vaccines.

References for Further Information on Childhood Immunizations

Online Resources

Center for Disease Control and Prevention (CDC) Websites

http://www.cdc.gov/vaccines

This is the home page for the Vaccines and Immunizations information section of the CDC. It provides links to a multitude of general information sources on all aspects of childhood immunizations. Separate links which can also be accessed from this home page include the following:

http://www.cdc.gov/vaccines/recs/schedules/default.htm
This CDC page links to all the current immunization schedules for children and adults.

http://www.cdc.gov/vaccines/vac-gen/default.htm
This section answers basic and common questions about vaccines.

http://www.cdc.gov/vaccines/vpd-vac/default.htm
Information in this section provides details on specific vaccines and vaccine-preventable diseases.

http://www.cdc.gov/vaccines/pubs/vis/default.htm
All CDC Vaccine Information Statements are available on this link.

http://www.cdc.gov/vaccinesafety
This is the CDC main site for vaccine safety, including information on autism and thimerosal.

Unless otherwise noted, the following websites provide general information for parents on many aspects of childhood immunizations.

http://www.cispimmunize.org
Immunization website for the AAP, American Academy of Pediatrics.

http://www.immunizationinfo.org/parents/index.cfm
National Network for Immunization Information, or NNii, website for parents.

http://www.vaccine.org
The Allied Vaccine Group, links to multiple websites on childhood immunizations.

http://www.vaccineinformation.org/children.asp
Vaccine information for parents of infants and children from the Immunization Action Coalition.

http://www.fda.gov/consumer/updates/kidsvaccines073107.pdf
Link to FDA Consumer Health Information, short guide entitled "A Parent's Guide to Kid's Vaccines."

http://www.chop.edu/consumer/jsp/division/generic.jsp?id=75697
The Children's Hospital of Philadelphia's Vaccine Education Center; the site provides many educational materials, including videos and DVDs.

The following websites provide information specific to vaccine safety, injury reporting, and compensation. (Please refer to excellent vaccine safety sites from the CDC, the AAP, and other sites noted previously).

http://www.vaccinesafety.edu
Johns Hopkins website on vaccine safety.

www.vaers.hhs.gov
Vaccine Adverse Event Reporting System (VAERS), discussed in questions 10, 22, and 23.

www.hrsa.gov/vaccinecompensation
National Vaccine Injury Compensation Program, discussed in question 23.

The following websites are parent-based and/or provide disease-specific information.

http://www.pkids.org
PKIDs, Parents of Kids with Infectious Diseases, provides information and support services for parents of children with certain types of infections.

http://www.nmaus.org
The National Meningitis Association (NMA) site provides education with a focus on meningococcal disease.

http://www.familiesfightingflu.org
Families Fighting Flu, for families and pediatricians who have lost a child to influenza, provides information about this specific infection and vaccine.

APPENDIX

Multimedia: Slide Series

http://www.cdc.gov/vaccines/vac-gen/ABCs/default.htm
This website provides the link to "The ABCs of Childhood Vaccines" slide series. The PowerPoint slide presentations cover information on vaccine safety, risks of not vaccinating, how vaccines work, natural immunity, and primary vaccinations.

Booklets

http://www.cdc.gov/vaccines/pubs/parents-guide/default.htm
This website provides a link to the 68-page booklet "The Parents' Guide to Childhood Immunizations," which discusses the common childhood diseases and vaccines. The booklet can be printed or a copy can be ordered online.

http://www3.niaid.nih.gov/topics/vaccines/PDF/undvacc.pdf
Website providing a link to the 52-page booklet "Understanding Vaccines," which is produced for parents by the U.S. Department of Health and Human Services, National Institute of Health and National Institute of Allergy and Infectious Diseases

Books

Vaccines: What You Should Know, Third Edition. Paul Offit, MD, and Louis Bell, MD. Wiley Publishers, 2003.

Vaccinating Your Child: Questions & Answers for the Concerned Parent. Sharon Humiston, MD, MPH, and Cynthia Good, Peachtree Publishers, 2000.

The Vaccine Book: Making the Right Decision for Your Child. Robert W. Sears, MD, FAAP, Little, Brown, and Co., 2007.

Do Vaccines Cause That?! A Guide for Evaluating Vaccine Safety Concerns. Martin G. Myers, Diego Pineda. i4ph, 2008.

100 Questions and Answers About Autism. Campion Quinn, M.D., Jones and Bartlett Publishers, 2006.

Glossary

A

Acetaminophen: A medicine often given to reduce pain and fever. Tylenol is a common brand name for this drug.

Active immunity: Protection of the body against disease or infection due to specific microorganisms. This type of immunity is acquired throughout your life, either after natural infections or immunization with vaccines.

Adaptive immunity: Another name for active immunity.

Adjuvants: Substances added to a vaccine to help make the immune response earlier, more potent or longer lasting. Aluminum salts are an example of an adjuvant used in a vaccine.

Advisory Committee on Immunization Practices (ACIP): A committee that gives official federal guidance and recommendations on the use of vaccines and the vaccine schedules in the United States.

AIDS: Acquired Immunodeficiency Syndrome, the final stage of HIV infection caused by virus-induced destruction of the immune system. There is currently no effective vaccine for the prevention of HIV.

American Academy of Family Physicians (AAFP): An organization of family physicians with a mission to promote the health of patients, families and communities. Like the AAP, the AAFP provides education and recommendations on vaccines and their use.

American Academy of Pediatrics (AAP): An organization of pediatricians who are advocates for children's health. A major activity of the AAP is to provide parents, healthcare providers, and the general public with education on many topics concerning children's health, including vaccines.

Anesthetic: A drug or substance which can produce decreased sensation or awareness. A topical anesthetic is applied to the skin to numb an area of skin prior to a procedure.

Anthrax: The disease caused by infection with the bacterium *Bacillus anthracis*. Most naturally acquired infections in people are skin infections, but severe infections of the lungs or stomach and intestines can occur. This bacterium has already been used in attempted bioterrorism activities. A vaccine is available for the prevention of anthrax but is not part of the recommended schedule of childhood vaccines.

Antibodies: Proteins made by immune cells in the body which help the body recognize microorganisms and fight off infection.

Antigens: Any substances foreign to the body that stimulate an immune response.

Attenuated vaccines: Vaccines which contain live but weakened microorganisms. The microorganisms in these vaccines are weakened by changing part of the germ so that it loses the properties that made it capable of causing disease.

Autism: A term often used to refer to a group of developmental disorders that affect the brain. (*See* Autism Spectrum Disorders).

Autism spectrum disorders (ASDs): A group of five related developmental and neurological disorders that affect the brain. Children with ASDs have a range of disabilities which may include difficulty in their ability to communicate, form relationships with others, and respond to their environment.

Avian influenza: A strain of influenza virus that has caused a large number of infections and death in birds in Southeast Asia and now other parts of the world. It is able to spread to humans and can cause severe disease. Avian Influenza is sometimes called the "bird flu."

B

Bacteremia: The presence of bacteria in the bloodstream. Bacteremia can occur with many types of infections, including bacterial pneumonia and bone infections.

Bacteria: Single-cell organisms that get nourishment from the environment. Many bacteria, such as *Streptococcus pneumoniae* and *Neisseria meningitidis*, can cause serious diseases in children. The singular form of bacteria is bacterium.

BCG (Bacille Calmette-Guerin): A vaccine for tuberculosis (TB) which is given to children in many countries with high rates of TB to try to prevent the disease in children. Two types of BCG are available in the United States, but the vaccine is not part of the routine immunization schedule.

Booster doses: Additional doses of a vaccine given to increase the immunity provided by that vaccine.

C

Centers for Disease Control and Prevention (CDC): An agency in the United States Department of Health and Social Services which works with local health departments and many other agencies to promote health as well as prevention and control of diseases in the United States.

Cervarix: A second HPV vaccine which is expected to be licensed for use in adolescent girls in late 2008 or 2009. This vaccine is made from HPV Types 16 and 18.

Cervical cancers: Cancer of the cervix (lower part of the uterus) or areas around the cervix. Cervical cancer can present with bleeding but often has no symptoms until the cancer is advanced. Pap smears are helpful in picking up early signs of these cancers. Human Papillomaviruses are associated with almost all cervical cancers.

Chickenpox: An illness with fever and a characteristic rash of pox on the skin. It is also called varicella, and is caused by infection with the Varicella-Zoster Virus.

Cirrhosis: Extensive scarring of the liver usually seen with chronic hepatitis. Cirrhosis can be caused by some types of liver infection, but also can result from long-standing alcohol abuse and other diseases.

Conjugate vaccine: A vaccine which has the microorganism (or part of the microorganism) attached to another compound which creates a better immune response.

Conjunctivitis: An infection of the conjunctiva, the inner surface of the eyelid and outer surface of the eye. Conjunctivitis can be caused by viruses or bacteria. The disease is also called "pink eye" or "red eye."

Croup: A respiratory illness, usually caused by a virus infection, which affects infants and young children. Children with croup often have a "barking cough" and a whistling sound (stridor) when taking a breath.

D

Diluent: The liquid used to dilute a vaccine to the right dose. The diluent is often water or saline.

Diphtheria: The disease caused by the bacterium *Corynebacterium diphtheriae*. The initial sore throat and fever progress to the development of a membrane in the back of the throat which can block the airway. Some patients may have heart failure or paralysis.

DT: A diphtheria-tetanus vaccine available for children under age 7 years who should not take the pertussis part of the vaccine due to concern arising from a prior reaction.

DTaP: The diphtheria, tetanus, acellular pertussis vaccine recommended for children at 2, 4, 6, 15–18 months, and 4–6 years of age.

Dysplastic lesions: Areas of skin or mucosa (e.g., in an area on the cervix seen on a pap smear) which show abnormal development or growth of cells or tissues.

E

EMLA cream: A type of topical anesthetic which is commonly used to numb the skin prior to certain medical procedures.

Encephalitis: An infection of the brain. Patients with encephalitis may have headache, fever, sensitivity of the eyes to light and even seizures. Many types of microorganisms can cause encephalitis, but usually it is due to an infection with a virus.

Epiglottitis: Inflammation of the epiglottis, which is the structure at the base of the tongue which stops food from entering the trachea (windpipe). Severe swelling can cause obstruction of the trachea and prevent breathing. In the past, *Haemophilus influenzae* type b was a common cause of epiglottitis.

Ethylmercury: A type of organic compound which contains mercury. Thimerosal, a vaccine preservative, contains ethylmercury.

Exemptions: In reference to vaccines, the term exemption denotes an official exception to the requirement for giving a child a vaccine. In many states, exemptions may be granted for medical, religious, or personal reasons.

F

Food and Drug Administration (FDA): The agency which is part of the United States Department of Health and Human Services which is responsible for the safety regulation of many items, including vaccines.

Food and Drug Administration Modernization Act: Legislation passed by the United States Congress which was geared to streamline the process of bringing safe and effective drugs, medical devices, and other therapies to the United States market. An amendment to the act in 1997 began the process of removing thimerosal from vaccines.

G

Gardasil: The first HPV vaccine approved in the United States. It helps protect against four types of HPV, including two which are at high risk of causing cervical cancer.

Guillain-Barre Syndrome: A disease of the nervous system which usually presents with weakness of the legs and spreads to the arms and face. The weakness often progresses to paralysis. The disease is usually triggered by an infection.

H

***Haemophilus influenzae* type b (Hib):** A bacterium which can cause a wide variety of infections in children, including pneumonia, bacteremia, meningitis, epiglottitis, and infection of the skin, joints, bones, and ears.

Hepatitis A Virus (HAV): A virus which can cause infection/inflammation of the liver. Hepatitis A is present in an infected person's stool, and is spread by direct contact or from contaminated food or water. This virus does not cause a chronic hepatitis.

Hepatitis B immune globulin: Specific antibody against Hepatitis B Virus. Often called "H-BIG," it is given with vaccine in certain circumstances to prevent transmission of this virus infection. The most common use is for infants born to a mother who has Hepatitis B.

Hepatitis B Virus (HBV): One of several viruses that can cause infection and/or inflammation of the liver. Transmission of this virus is usually by exposure to infected blood or body fluids.

Hepatitis C Virus (HCV): Another virus which can cause infection and/or inflammation of the liver. Like Hepatitis B Virus, infection is usually from exposure to infected blood or body fluids. There is no current vaccine which can prevent Hepatitis C.

Herd immunity: Protection of unimmunized people from a specific infection or disease which is obtained by immunizing a large percentage of people in families and the community.

Human Immunodeficiency Virus (HIV): The virus that causes AIDS. Although significant efforts have been made to find an effective vaccine, there is currently no vaccine available to prevent infection with HIV.

Human Papillomavirus (HPV): A common virus which causes various types of warts, including genital warts. Warts on the skin are not usually problematic, but some types of HPV causing genital warts can lead to cervical cancer.

Hygiene: Practices such as washing hands, bathing, and brushing teeth which are associated with general cleanliness and ensuring good health.

I

Ibuprofen: A medicine often given to reduce pain and fever. Advil and Motrin are common brand names for this drug.

Immune system: The cells, glands, and fluids throughout the body which work together to fight microorganisms. The job of the immune system is to react to the microorganisms to help fight or prevent infection.

Immunity: Protection of the body from either a disease or from infection by a microorganism.

Immunization: The process of giving a vaccine to someone in order to bring about immunity. This is sometimes also called vaccination.

Inactivated polio vaccine (IPV): The current polio vaccine used in the

United States. The vaccine has killed virus from each of the three types of poliovirus.

Influenza: Often called "the flu," this is the disease caused by one of the influenza viruses. The illness often starts with cold-like symptoms such as sore throat, headache, fever, and muscle aches, but may be complicated by pneumonia and other serious complications.

Innate immunity: Part of the general response of the body which provides non-specific protection from the presence of an invading germ. The skin, stomach lining, nose, and other body surfaces provide part of this protection. This is also called natural immunity.

Institute of Medicine: A non-governmental agency which provides health information to policy-makers, healthcare professionals, and the general public.

Intussusception: A blockage or twisting of the intestine which can be life-threatening. Although intussusception can happen at any age, it most commonly occurs in the first year of life. The vaccine RotaShield was taken off the market due to concerns of increased risk of intussusception.

Investigational New Drug (IND): An official designation by the United States Food and Drug Administration (FDA) for an experimental vaccine that has not yet been approved for marketing. The IND designation is required before the vaccine can be transported across state lines.

Iron Lungs: Machines used in the past to treat people with severe polio who were unable to breathe without assistance. With severe polio, the muscles needed for breathing could be paralyzed, and patients would die without the use of a machine to help them breathe.

J

Japanese Encephalitis: A disease caused by the Japanese Encephalitis Virus. It is prevalent in areas of Asia and Australia, and is transmitted to humans via the bite of infected mosquitoes. Infection with the virus can cause encephalitis. A killed vaccine is available for travelers to areas where the virus is commonly found.

Jaundice: A yellow color of the skin and eyes, usually seen in people who have hepatitis, an inflammation or infection of the liver.

K

Killed vaccines: Vaccines which contain only killed or inactivated microorganisms. These vaccines cannot cause infection in the recipient because the germs are not living.

L

Lyme disease: An infectious disease caused by a microorganism called *Borrelia burgdorferi*. The hallmark of

Lyme disease is a characteristic rash, although non-specific symptoms may develop and untreated infections may lead to chronic complications. Infection occurs from the bite of an infected deer tick.

LYMErix: A vaccine against Lyme disease approved for use in the United States in 1998, but soon taken off the market. Currently there is no vaccine available in the United States to prevent Lyme disease.

M

Measles: The disease caused by the virus of the same name. Children with measles have a runny nose, conjunctivitis, cough, fever, and a characteristic red rash. Complications of pneumonia and encephalitis can be severe.

Meningitis: Infection of the lining or membranes around the brain. Children with meningitis may have fever, stiff neck, headache, and other non-specific symptoms. Meningitis can be caused by various bacteria and viruses.

Meningococcus: *Neisseria meningitidis,* a bacterium which can cause life-threatening bloodstream infection and meningitis.

Methylmercury: One type of organic compound which contains mercury.

Microorganisms: A more formal word for germs, things too small to be seen by the naked eye which may

cause infections. Bacteria and viruses are common types of microorganisms.

Mitochondrial disorder: A specific type of disease which can affect the brain and can be associated with various neurologic symptoms which become more severe as the child ages.

MMR vaccine: The live virus vaccine given to prevent measles, mumps, and rubella.

Multiple sclerosis (MS): A chronic, progressive disease that involves the brain, spinal cord, and other parts of the central nervous system. MS is considered an autoimmune disease.

Mumps: A disease caused by the mumps virus. Children may have cold-like symptoms such as fever, headache, and muscle aches, but the hallmark of the infection is swelling of salivary glands such as the parotid gland.

N

National Childhood Vaccine Injury Act (NCVIA): Legislation passed in 1986 to help protect vaccine makers from the financial liability involved with lawsuits arising from vaccine injury. Part of this act was the creation of the National Vaccine Injury Compensation Program (NVICP), which created a claim system for compensating victims of vaccine-related injuries.

Natural immunity: Part of the general response of the body to the presence of an invading germ which provides non-specific protection. The skin, stomach lining, nose, and other body surfaces provide part of this protection. This is also called innate immunity.

Necrotizing fasciitis: A severe infection involving the skin and deeper tissues which is often caused by the same streptococcus bacterium that causes "strep throat." Children with chickenpox have an increased risk of developing necrotizing fasciitis and other milder forms of skin infection.

Neisseria meningitidis: A bacterium which can cause life-threatening bloodstream infection and meningitis. It is also called meningococcus.

Nosodes: A class of remedies used by some practitioners of homeopathy. The substances are prepared from dilutions of material obtained from a person with a specific disease.

O

Oral Polio Vaccine (OPV): A live polio vaccine no longer used in the United States but still in use in other countries. The OPV was taken by mouth. The inactivated polio vaccine, a killed vaccine, is currently used in the United States.

P

Parotid gland: A salivary gland (which makes saliva in the mouth) which is located at the jaw line just below the ear. The parotid gland can become swollen in children with mumps.

Passive immunity: Protection of the body from disease or infection which develops when a person is given antibodies. Passive immunity is acquired by infants when antibodies are passed across the placenta during pregnancy and via breast feeding.

Pathogen: A microorganism which can cause infection or disease.

Pertussis: The disease caused by infection with the bacterium *Bordetella pertussis*. The hallmark of the disease, which is also called whooping cough, is long, paroxysms of coughing, occasionally ending with a "whoop."

Pneumococcus: Another name for the bacterium *Streptococcus pneumoniae*, a bacterium associated with many types of infections in children.

Pneumovax: The pneumococcal vaccine for use in older children and adults. Due to the type of vaccine, it is not effective in infants and children younger than age 2. Prevnar is the pneumococcal vaccine used in infants and young children.

Polio: The disease caused by the virus of the same name. Most people with polio do not have symptoms, but signs and symptoms could range from sore throat, fever and runny nose with occasional pain in the neck, back, or legs to severe leg pains followed by paralysis.

Preservatives: Substances added to a vaccine to help the vaccine remain sterile.

Prevnar: The killed pneumococcal vaccine used in infants and young children. The vaccine contains the top 7 types of the bacterium which cause most invasive disease in young children. It is recommended for ages 2, 4, 6, and 12–15 months.

R

Rabies: A severe disease of the brain and nervous system caused by rabies virus infection. The disease is almost always fatal. Bites from an infected bat currently cause most of the human cases of rabies in the United States.

Relenza (Zanamavir): A medicine used for both treatment and prevention of influenza. Relenza is dispensed in a powder form in an inhaler. It is approved for use in children older than age 7 for treatment and older than age 5 for prevention of influenza.

Rotarix: A rotavirus vaccine approved in 2008 for use in young infants.

RotaShield: The first rotavirus vaccine approved for use in the United States. The vaccine was taken off the market due to concerns about the association of use of this vaccine with a severe intestinal disease called intussusception.

RotaTeq: A rotavirus vaccine approved in 2006 for use in young infants.

Rotavirus: A common, highly contagious virus that is an important cause of severe diarrhea in children.

Rubella: A disease caused by the rubella virus. The disease is also called German measles or three-day measles. Rubella can cause fever, mild rash, swollen glands in the neck, and sometimes arthritis. Infection during pregnancy can lead to various birth defects in infants.

S

Sexually-transmitted disease (STD): Any infection or disease which is transmitted to someone else by unprotected sex. Common sexually-transmitted diseases include Human Papillomavirus infections, HIV, syphilis, genital herpes, chlamydia, and gonorrhea.

Shingles: Also called zoster, this disease is a recurrence of disease with the virus that causes chickenpox (varicella). Unlike chickenpox, shingles usually occurs later in life and presents with rash in only a small area of the skin.

Smallpox: A disease characterized by high fever, spots in the mouth, and a rash with classic "pox" lesions. This very contagious and often severe disease was the first virus infection eradicated from the world through the use of vaccines.

Stabilizers: Substances added to a vaccine to help the vaccine stay potent even with changes in temperature, humidity, light, or acidity. MSG (monosodium glutamate) and albumin (protein) are two examples of stabilizers used in vaccines.

State Children's Health Insurance Program (SCHIP): A program, also known as Title XXI, which helps states to expand health insurance coverage for uninsured children so that more children may be eligible for the Vaccines for Children program.

Streptococcus pneumoniae: A common bacterium which causes many types of infections in children. Diseases associated with this bacterium include meningitis, pneumonia, bacteremia, sinus and ear infections, conjunctivitis (type of eye infection), and other serious diseases.

Subunit vaccine: One of the four basic types of vaccines. It is named "subunit" because only part of the microorganism is present in the vaccine.

Sudden infant death syndrome (SIDS): A term used to denote the sudden and unexplained death of an apparently healthy infant aged one month to one year.

T

Tamiflu (Oseltamivir): A medicine used for both treatment and prevention of influenza. Tamiflu is available in capsules or liquid, and can be used in children older than 12 months of age.

Td: The tetanus-diphtheria vaccine given to children older than age 7 years for booster vaccines as needed. To avoid adverse reactions, Td has a smaller amount of the diphtheria and a normal amount of the tetanus.

Tdap: A combination vaccine against tetanus, diphtheria, and acellular pertussis approved in 2005 for use in teenagers and some adults. This vaccine has the normal amount of tetanus with reduced amounts of both diphtheria and pertussis.

Tetanus: A disease which affects the nervous system and is caused by the bacterium *Clostridium tetani*. Also called "lockjaw," tetanus in known for muscle spasms which occur in jaw muscles (causing "lockjaw" or trismus), but also in muscles of the neck, arms, legs, and most muscle groups.

Tetanus immune globulin (TIG): A preparation which contains antibody to tetanus. TIG can be given to anyone who is at risk of getting tetanus. It provides protection faster but only for a short time, so a tetanus vaccine is usually given at the same time as TIG.

Thimerosal: A vaccine preservative which contains ethylmercury. Thimerosal was used extensively in the past, but is currently present in small amounts in only a few vaccines.

Toxoids: Types of vaccines which are made from inactive toxic compounds. The vaccines for tetanus and diphtheria are examples of toxoids.

Tuberculosis (TB): The disease caused by the bacterium *Mycobacterium tuberculosis*. Although many think of TB as a disease affecting only the lungs, many parts of the body can be affected by this disease. BCG (Bacille

Calmette-Guerin) is a vaccine for TB which is given in many countries but not routinely used in the United States.

Typhoid fever: An acute, life-threatening illness with fever caused by the bacterium *Salmonella typhi*. Two types of vaccines are available for use for the prevention of infection with this bacterium.

V

Vaccination: The process of giving a vaccine to someone in order to bring about immunity. This is also called immunization.

Vaccine: A substance that teaches the body to recognize and defend itself against a disease-causing germ.

Vaccine Adverse Event Reporting System (VAERS): A national reporting system in the United States that accepts reports from the public (doctors, nurses, parents, anyone) regarding adverse events associated with any vaccine licensed in the United States.

Vaccine-Associated Paralytic Polio (VAPP): A type of polio which was associated with use of the older live virus vaccine which is no longer used in the United States.

Vaccine Information Statement (VIS): A form developed by the Center for Disease Control and Prevention (CDC) which provides information on the risks and benefits of individual vaccines.

Vaccine Registries: Computerized information systems which collect vaccine histories and help ensure timely administration of vaccines for children.

Vaccine Safety Datalink (VSD): A project of the CDC and eight large managed care organizations which monitors a large population of patients in the United States to assess vaccine safety.

Vaccines for Children (VFC) Program: A federal program which helps families who have difficulty paying for vaccines to obtain vaccines for their children. Children through age 18 years of age who are Medicaid eligible, uninsured, an American Indian or Alaskan Native, or who are underinsured are eligible for the program.

Varicella: An illness with fever and a characteristic rash of pox on the skin. It is also called chickenpox, and is caused by infection with the Varicella-Zoster Virus.

Varivax: The live virus vaccine used to try to prevent chickenpox (varicella).

Viruses: Types of germs, or microorganisms, which are "non-living," and need to live in other cells to survive. Viruses are the most common germs which cause infections in children.

W

Warts: Common warts are small, often rough, lesions on the skin which are frequently seen on the hands or feet. Warts are caused by

Human Papillomavirus infection. Genital infection with this virus is also very frequent. Some types of HPV associated with genital warts can cause cervical cancer.

Y

Yellow fever: A disease caused by Yellow fever virus. This virus is found mainly in parts of Africa and South America and is transmitted to humans via infected mosquitoes. Yellow fever ranges from an illness like influenza to severe hepatitis and hemorrhagic fever. A live virus vaccine is available for travelers to areas where this virus is commonly found.

Z

Zostavax: A vaccine given to people to prevent the development of shingles (zoster). Currently it is used only in adults more than 60 years old and is not a childhood vaccine.

Index